Paleo Desserts: Sugar Detox:

Gluten Free for Paleo Baking & Paleo Beginners; Detox Cleanse to Heal the Sugar Addiction, Lose Belly Fat & Increase Energy

Emma Rose

Paleo Desserts

Satisfy Your Sweet Tooth With Over 100 Quick and Easy Paleo Dessert Recipes and Paleo Baking Recipes

Emma Rose

Table Of Contents

Introduction   1

Chapter 1 - Brief History of Paleo Free Diet   4

Chapter 2 - Chocolatiest at its best!   7

Chapter 3 - Baked Chocolate Goodness   28

Chapter 4 - Drinks For Desserts   42

Chapter 5 - Kids At Work   45

Chapter 6 - Other Goodies   48

Bonus   96

Conclusion   105

Preview of Next Book   106

Introduction

I want to thank you for purchasing this book!

This book contains 100 Paleo dessert and baking recipes on how to prepare delectable desserts without sacrificing your health.

All my life I've had a sweet tooth. I would even go as far as to say that I had a sugar addiction! Over the last few years my sugar addiction got worse: I had dessert multiple times a day and every day (I guess being a Foods teacher didn't help much). I would joke with people by telling them that I had my servings of vegetables for the day in chocolate...except, I still didn't have the vegetables. It got pretty bad. I knew I hated eating that much dessert but I couldn't stop. I would eat one Ferrero Rocher and then go back for another. As I walked back to the treats, I would pass the mirror and think to myself, "I don't need to have this chocolate. But, ah, what the heck, I don't care." In the end, I'd have about 6 Ferrero Rocher in addition to the other treats I had earlier that day.

Finally, I had to take the huge tray of Ferrero Rocher to school to give to my students on Valentine's Day. There was no way I could eat the other 30 myself. Eating all this sugar caused a huge war within me. I knew that my extreme sugar eating was unhealthy for me but I didn't want to stop. I loved it too much. As a result, I wrestled between the ideal of where I wanted to be and the reality of where I was. I knew I had the discipline to say no to other things, so why couldn't I say no to chocolate?

I eventually came to the point where I was starting to get fed up with not feeling well. I had a lot of chronic pain in my neck and I was constantly tired. I knew that sugar was irritating the problem and causing inflammation in my body. At was starting to reach the breaking point. Ultimately, I chose to go off of sugar for at least three weeks to break the habit I had created for myself. It was seriously a miracle to stay consistent with my goal because I really didn't want to give up my favorite desserts.

Shortly after my decision to go off of sugar, I had a miscarriage. Experiencing the loss catapulted me into a massive journey to find health and proper nutrition. I did a live blood analysis with a naturopath to discover what was contributing to the terrible ways I was feeling. Seeing all the garbage I had in my blood forced me to go off of dairy, corn, oats, and wheat. I was left wondering, "What the heck am I going to eat? That stuff is in everything!"

Consequently, I stumbled upon the Paleo Free Diet. It was the most relevant diet to what I was trying to accomplish. I was able to find things to eat for breakfast, lunch and dinner. But desserts were a whole other story. I felt like something was missing and I couldn't put my finger on it. The best I could come up with was apple slices dipped in almond butter: hardly satisfying. Paleo desserts ended up being the by-product of my search to find something, anything that I could enjoy.

I encourage you to make that switch to healthier and happier desserts with the hundred delicious and irresistible recipes presented in this book. You don't need to follow the same extremity that I did. But if you are taking the Paleo Free Diet seriously, then you may find the same void of sweets in your life too. Cutting out all the processed foods and going back to the basics really does clear up the body and help it function better.

I've seen the changes in my own life as hard as it's been to make those changes. You, too, can make the changes necessary and still have your sweets along the way!

Thank you again for purchasing this book. I hope you enjoy the recipes. Experiment with them and make substitutions to suit your needs.

With gratitude,

Emma Rose

Chapter 1

Brief History of Paleo Free Diet

The Sweet Effects

Why do you love sweet food? Why do you crave for more dessert so much? Your anatomy would tell you that sweet foods would cause the release of dopamine in the part of the brain that is associated with motivation and reward. Not only that, but studies show that sweets also produce an increased level of serotonin. Serotonin gives you that feeling of happiness and wellbeing. That's why it is better to give a box of chocolates when you want a person to be in a good mood.

Unfortunately, the quote, "You can't have your cake and eat it too," applies here. The negative effects that sugar brings are common knowledge. One of the top most common diseases is diabetes. People are well aware of diabetes and its complications. As a result, when you intensely crave for that delicious dessert, you try to control your urges and settle for nothing instead. However, that only works if your self-control is in good condition. More often than not, people would rather risk the medical condition and eat that sweet thing with all their heart.

I have had many slip ups in my own life. I went two months without chocolate...can you believe it? Then Easter came. I found that if I gave myself an inch, I would take a mile. Eating chocolate quickly got out of control. I rebelled because I was strict for so long. You may find yourself in the same situation and find it hard to balance the sugar cravings. Once the sugar cravings are there, your body craves more and then a vicious cycle begins.

What is Paleo Free Diet?
This is when my book comes to the rescue! You can have your cake and eat it too, literally. And not just cake only, but lots more!

Paleo has been known by many names such as the cavemen diet, stone age diet and hunter-gatherer diet, to name a few. The concept behind this diet follows that of the Paleolithic era before the development of agriculture. This type of diet is still very young, only less than fifty years. However, more in depth research and studies are being conducted to increase the information and knowledge of this diet.

The results of previous studies on the Paleo Free Diet reveal an improvement in health to the people involved. This is attributed to the fact that no processed foods and additives are included. Foods that were not available during the Paleolithic time such as dairy products, salt, sugar and grains are also not included in the preparation of the Paleo Free Diet. These ingredients are often though to cause some diseases such as hypertension, diabetes, strokes, obesity and other heart problems.

You will notice that sugar shows up in the form of honey, maple syrup or chocolate. It can be argued that these sources are natural compared to the refined sugar which is a by-product of our industrialization and modern world. The history of chocolate dates back to the ancient Mayans who used the cacao pods as a form of currency. You can be the judge as to whether you want to include these foods in your diet. When it comes to chocolate, I prefer organic fair trade chocolate made from cacao powder. Cacao powder is more unrefined and unprocessed compared to cocoa powder.

In this book you will find a hundred recipes to satisfy your sweet tooth by using these prehistoric ingredients free of additives and processed foods. Are you ready to satisfy your cravings? Here are the simple and easy to follow recipes that you would surely fall in love with.

Chapter 2 – Chocolatiest at its Best!

Who doesn't love chocolate? Here are over 30 recipes with chocolate as the main ingredient. Dairy free chocolates are preferred. And half of these recipes do not even need an oven to create them.

Brownie Magic

This recipe is super quick and only involves 3 common ingredients: cocoa powder, dates and walnuts.

Ingredients:
1 tablespoon cocoa powder
1 cup dates (softened in water first)
1 cup walnuts

Procedure:
Add the three ingredients into a blender and blend until smooth. Adjust the cocoa powder to taste. Once satisfied, roll the mixture into small balls. You'll have a brownie ready to munch anytime – morning, noon or night. Keep stored in refrigerator.

The 3 C's Dessert

These basic ingredients start with the letter C – chocolates, coffee and coconut butter.

Ingredients:
½ cup coconut butter, melted
1 tablespoon ground coffee
3 tablespoon 100% cocoa powder
½ teaspoon honey

Procedure:
Combine and mix thoroughly the coconut butter, ground coffee, cocoa powder, and honey. Lightly grease an ice cube tray with coconut oil. Then spoon the mixture and place them in the ice cube tray. Leave the ice cube tray in the freezer for 5 hours. Remove the tray from the freezer 15 minutes before serving.

Dairy Free Delight Part 1

The main base:

Ingredients:
2 cans (24 ounces) pure coconut milk
¼ cup cocoa powder
¼ teaspoon sweetener of choice
2 ounces unsweetened chocolate
1.5 tablespoon pure vanilla extract

Procedure:
Heat the coconut milk and cocoa powder in a medium saucepan on low-medium heat. Add the sweetener of your choice, unsweetened chocolate and pure vanilla extract. Allow the chocolate to melt and remove from heat. Let it cool and then place in the refrigerator for at least four hours. Remove from refrigerator and serve cool.

Dairy Free Delight Part 2

Follow the same procedure in Part 1 but instead of serving it as it is, put the cooled mixture into an ice cream maker. Follow the manufacturer's instruction. Afterwards, you may want to top it with fresh fruit. Serve immediately. Or you may want to try Part 3.

Dairy Free Delight Part 3

A different version of Part 2 would be instead of serving it, put it back in the freezer for another hour (right after the coffee and talks would be great). As a result, the ice cream would be firmer.

Dairy Free Delight Part 4

Place the cooled mixture into popsicle molds and freeze for 4 hours. This treat is great for kids.

Chunky Choco

Ingredients:
6 ounces unsweetened chocolate
½ teaspoon vanilla
1/8 teaspoon sweetener of choice

Procedure:
Melt unsweetened chocolate using a double boiler. Make sure that the chocolate is completely melted. Remove from heat and continue stirring the chocolate while you add vanilla and sweetener of your choice. Place in a pan and let it set in the refrigerator for 30-45 minutes. You can cut into squares or let the kids design their own chunky chocolate.

Apple Chocolate on a Stick

Insert a stick through the core of the apple (children, let the adults do this). Melt a bar of dark chocolate. When the chocolate is fully melted, dip the apple. Put in the refrigerator for 20 minutes to set. You can eat it as is or let the kids be more creative and add some toppings prior to placing it on the refrigerator.

Sixty Seconds Dessert

Ingredients:
2 tablespoon coconut milk
1 tablespoon unsweetened cocoa powder
2 tablespoon coconut butter
¾ teaspoon pure vanilla extract
2 servings of sweetener of choice, to taste

Procedure:
In a small bowl, add the following ingredients: coconut milk, unsweetened cocoa powder, coconut butter, pure vanilla extract and sweetener. Use the back of the spoon to blend it until smooth.

Dark Chocolate Pudding

Ingredients:
1 egg, beaten
½ ripe avocado
¼ cup coconut milk
2 tablespoon cacao powder
1 tablespoon coffee
1 pinch salt
1 pinch cinnamon powder
1 scoop vanilla flavored whey protein powder
0.35 ounces raw hazelnuts
2 tablespoon unsweetened shredded coconut

Procedure:
Put beaten egg, avocado and coconut milk into a blender or food processor and blend until smooth. Add cacao powder, coffee, salt, cinnamon powder and vanilla flavored whey protein powder. Blend until smooth again. Add raw hazelnuts and unsweetened shredded coconut and let it spin until the hazelnuts are turned into small pieces. Serve immediately or refrigerate before serving. You can top it with more tiny pieces hazelnut if you want.

10 Minutes No-Bake Cookies

You could also call this the salted caramel chocolate chunk cookies

Ingredients:
1 ½ cups sugar (try date or coconut sugar)
½ cup coconut milk
½ cup coconut oil
2 teaspoon vanilla extract
½ teaspoon sea salt
1 cup flake coconut
2/3 cup chocolate chunks or chips

Procedure:
In a saucepan, combine the following ingredients: sugar, coconut milk and coconut oil. Constantly stir while you bring it to boil. After 2-3 minutes of boiling (again, stir continuously- you don't want caramel to stick), remove from heat and add vanilla extract, sea salt and flake coconut. Add chocolate chunks or chips and stir softly. Set it in a pan and let it set for 2-3 hours. You can cut the cookies into the shapes that you like.

Chocolate Madness

Make chocolate cookies using the 10 Minutes No Bake Cookies. Place on a plate and add a small scoop of homemade chocolate ice cream. Top with chocolate chips. Serve!

Choco Fudge

Ingredients:
¼ cup cocoa butter
¼ cup coconut oil
½ cup coconut butter
1 tablespoon honey
¼ serving of sweetener of choice, to taste
¼ cup cocoa powder
1 teaspoon vanilla

Procedure:
In a pan with low heat, melt the cocoa butter. Add the cocoa butter, coconut oil and coconut butter. Use a whisk to mix. Add the honey, sweetener, cocoa powder and vanilla and gently whisk. Make sure that everything is properly mixed. There should be no lumps. Do not overheat. Place in an 8" by 8" pan lined with parchment paper and refrigerate for 1-2 hours. Cut according to your preference.

Chocolate Custard Delight

Ingredients:
1 can coconut milk
1 cup dark chocolate
1 teaspoon vanilla

Procedure:
In a saucepan over low-medium heat, combine coconut milk and dark chocolate. Mix with a whisk until chocolate is melted. Add vanilla. Pour into smaller glasses and let it set in the refrigerator. Top it with fresh fruit.

Strawberry Coated Chocolates

Melt a bar of dark chocolate by using a double broiler. Dip as many strawberries as you want. Serve immediately.

Cookie Topper

Ingredients:
3 tablespoon coconut milk
2 tablespoon coconut cream, concentrate
½ tablespoon pure vanilla extract
3 tablespoon cacao powder
3 servings of sweetener of choice, to taste

Procedure:
In a bowl, combine coconut milk and coconut cream concentrate. Add pure vanilla extract, cacao powder and sweetener. Whisk until the mixture is very creamy. Place on top of any homemade cookie. Add ice cream if you like.

Choco Fruit Dip

Ingredients:
1 cup coconut
1 teaspoon vanilla
2 ripe bananas
2 teaspoon coconut flour
1 ½ tablespoon unsweetened cocoa powder

Procedure:
Place into a food processor or blender the following ingredients: coconut, vanilla, bananas and coconut flour. Blend until smooth. Add the unsweetened cocoa powder. Serve with a platter of strawberries or apples.

Black Forest Shake

Ingredients:
1 cup pitted cherries
2 tablespoon unsweetened cocoa powder
1 cup coconut milk

Procedure:
Place in a blender pitted cherries, unsweetened cocoa powder, coconut milk. Whir until smooth. Top with toasted shredded coconut.

Choco Thickshake

Ingredients:
4 dried dates
½ banana
1/3 cup hazelnuts
1 teaspoon honey
1 tablespoon cocoa powder
1 tablespoon cacao powder
1 cup coconut milk
3-4 ice cubes
¼ cup strong coffee

Procedure:
Place in a blender the following ingredients: dried dates, banana, hazelnuts, honey, cocoa powder, cacao powder, coconut milk, ice, and strong coffee. Blend until smooth.

Minty Chocolate Shake

Ingredients:
1 tablespoon maple syrup
8 fresh mint leaves
1 ½ tablespoon cocoa powder
1 cup coconut cream
3-4 ice cubes

Procedure:
Combine and blend the following: maple syrup, mint leaves, cocoa powder, coconut cream and ice cubes. Blend until smooth.

Strawberry with Chocolate Chips Ice Cream

Ingredients:
5-7 frozen strawberries
½ cup coconut milk
1 teaspoon vanilla extract

Procedure:
Blend frozen strawberries, coconut milk and vanilla extract. Place in the freezer for one hour. Top with chocolate chips. Then it's ready to be served!

Yummy Pudding

Ingredients:
1 egg
¼ cup coconut milk
2 tablespoon cacao powder
1 scoop chocolate flavored protein powder
1 pinch sea salt
1 pinch cinnamon powder

Procedure:
Blend until smooth the following: egg, coconut milk, cacao powder, chocolate flavored protein powder, sea salt and cinnamon powder. Refrigerate for at least 30 minutes. Top with nuts, if you wish.

Chocolate-Raspberry Layered Delight

In a small glass, pour melted chocolate. Place ¼ cup raspberries. Pour melted chocolate again and a spoonful of almond butter. Place 2 sliced bananas on top and finish with a melted chocolate.

Chocolate Shot

Ingredients:
3 tablespoon coconut milk
1 ½ tablespoon cocoa powder
½ teaspoon vanilla
1 serving of sweetener

Procedure:
Prepare this dessert by adding coconut milk, cocoa powder, vanilla and sweetener. Blend until smooth. Place is a small shot cup.

Apple and Honey Chocolate Coated Dessert

Insert a stick to the apple's core. Lightly brush the apple all over with honey. Melt a bar of dark chocolate. Dip the apple with honey on the chocolate. Let it set in the refrigerator.

Caramelized Banana on Chocolate Ice Cream

Make a homemade chocolate ice cream. Place in the freezer. Over low heat, place 2 pieces bananas, peeled and cut into small pieces, into the pan. Add 1 tablespoon maple syrup or honey until it thickens a little. Remove from heat, and allow to cool for several minutes. Place on top of the ice cream.

Chocolate Filled Peaches
Melt a bar of your favorite Paleo dark chocolate bar. Get 3-5 peaches, peeled and cut into halves. Remove the inner core and fill it with the melted chocolate instead. Set in the refrigerator for 30 minutes.

Banana and Chocolate

Get a ripe banana and quarter it but do not remove the peel. Pour a tablespoon of melted chocolate over the banana. Add chocolate chips on the side.

Strawberry And Chocolate Combo

Using a double broiler, melt a bar of dark chocolate. Cut the strawberry into halves and core the center. Place the melted chocolate into the center.

Minty Black Forest Shake

This is a combination of the Black Forest Shake Place and Minty Chocolate Shake.

Ingredients:
2 tablespoon unsweetened cocoa powder
1 cup pitted cherries
1 cup coconut milk
5-6 pieces mint leaves

Procedure:
Blend the following: unsweetened cocoa powder, pitted cherries, coconut milk and mint leaves. Whirl until smooth. You may serve it with nuts or chocolate chips on top.

Coffee and Coconut Sweets

Ingredients:
½ cup coconut butter
2 tablespoon 100% cocoa powder
1 tablespoon ground coffee
½ teaspoon honey
1 tablespoon coconut flakes

Procedure:
Melt coconut butter and add 100% cocoa powder, ground coffee, honey, and coconut flakes. Mix well. Evenly grease coconut oil in the cups of the ice cube tray and place the mixture into each cup. Freeze for 4 hours and take out of the freezer 15 minutes before serving.

Although there were no ovens yet during the Stone Age, all the ingredients here are prehistoric.

Choco Cookies

Ingredients:
1 ½ cups almond flour
¼ teaspoon baking soda
¼ teaspoon sea salt
½ cup chocolate chips

2 tablespoon coconut oil
½ teaspoon vanilla
½ cup maple syrup
1 egg

Procedure:
In a bowl, combine the following ingredients: almond flour, baking soda, sea salt and chocolate chips. In a separate bowl, mix the following: coconut oil, vanilla, maple syrup and egg. Combine the two mixtures and let the batter sit in the refrigerator for 30 minutes.

While waiting for the batter, line the baking sheet with parchment paper. The oven should be preheated to 350°F. Place the batter onto the sheet according to the size of the cookies that you like. Bake for 5 minutes. Take the baking sheet out of the oven and flatten each cookie. Put the baking sheet back for another 5 minutes. Let it cool before serving.

Beets and Banana Brownie

Ingredients:
2 red cooked beets
2 eggs
½ cup chocolate protein powder
½ cup unsweetened cacao powder
2 bananas
1/3 cup almonds
1 teaspoon baking powder

Procedure:
Preheat the oven to 325°F. Combine the following in the blender and blend – red cooked beets, eggs, chocolate protein powder, unsweetened cacao powder, bananas, 1 almonds, and baking powder. Pour into an 8" x 8" lightly greased pan. Bake for 30 minutes.

Classic Chocolate-Strawberry Bars

Ingredients:
2 ¼ cups almond flour
½ cup coconut sugar
½ teaspoon baking powder
6 tablespoon flaxseed meal
¼ teaspoon sea salt
2/3 cups arrowroot powder

6 tablespoon coconut oil, melted
3 tablespoon coconut milk
2 teaspoon vanilla extract

½ cup dark chocolate chips
½ cup fresh cut strawberries
1 tablespoon fresh lemon juice
Handful chopped almonds (optional)

Procedure:
Preheat the oven to 350°F. Combine in a bowl almond flour, coconut sugar, baking powder, flaxseed meal, sea salt and arrowroot powder. In a separate bowl, whisk the following: melted coconut oil, coconut milk and vanilla extract. Mix together the wet and dry ingredients using a gloved hand. This will form soft dough. Take note not to over mix this.

Reserve ½ cup of dough to be used later. Place the remaining dough on an 8" x 8" baking pan lined with parchment paper. Top with ½ cup dark chocolate chips. Cover the chips with fresh cut strawberries. Drizzle with fresh lemon juice and then drizzle with the extra dough plus an extra handful of almonds. Bake the dough for 20 minutes then lower the heat to 325°F and then bake for another 10 minutes. It should turn into a beautiful golden color crumble bar. Cut and serve.

Choco Chip Cookies

Ingredients:
¾ cup almond flour
¼ cup coconut flour
1/4 teaspoon plus 2 servings of sweetener
½ cup chopped nuts
2 teaspoon baking powder

5 tablespoon coconut butter
1 teaspoon vanilla extract
½ tablespoon honey

Procedure:
Preheat the oven to 350°F. Combine all the dry ingredients in a bowl: almond flour, coconut flour, plus sweeteners, chopped nuts and baking powder. In a separate bowl, combine all the wet ingredients: coconut butter, vanilla extract and honey. Combine the wet and dry ingredients until a dough is formed.

Using a small scooper, shape the dough into balls and place them three inches away from each other on the parchment paper baking pan. Flatten them with your hand and bake. Oven time will vary but it is usually around 10-15 minutes or until brown. Serve immediately.

Fudgy Bars

Ingredients:
2 cups almond flour
½ cup flaxseed meal
½ teaspoon sea salt
½ cup coconut sugar
2 teaspoon cinnamon powder (optional)
1/3 cup chocolate chunks

1 egg
1 tablespoon vanilla extract
1 cup pumpkin puree

Procedure:
Preheat the oven to 350°F. Mix the following ingredients in a bowl – almond flour, flaxseed meal, sea salt, coconut sugar, cinnamon powder and chocolate chunks. In a separate bowl, whisk egg, vanilla extract and pumpkin puree. Mix the dry and wet ingredients. Be careful not to over mix because it causes extra oiliness. Spread into a lightly greased baking pan. Bake around 25 minutes.

Choco Banana Surprise

Ingredients:
2 over ripe bananas
3 beaten eggs
¼ cup coconut oil
½ cup almond butter
3 tablespoon coconut flour
½ teaspoon baking soda
¼ teaspoon salt
1/3 cup mini chocolate chips

Procedure:
Preheat the oven to 350°F. Mash bananas. Add eggs, coconut oil, almond butter, coconut flour, baking soda and salt. Mix thoroughly until a batter is formed. Fold in mini chocolate chips. Pour the batter into the baking pan and spread evenly. Bake for 15-20 minutes. Let it cool. Cut into squares.

Choco Cake

Ingredients:
7.8 ounces dark chocolate
5 egg, separated
4.2 ounces coconut sugar
5.3 ounces grams almond meal
1 shot coffee
¾ cup raspberries

Procedure:
Preheat the oven to 350°F. Melt dark chocolate and let cool. Set aside. In a bowl, whisk egg whites and add coconut sugar. Fold half of this mixture into the egg yolks. Continue to fold the egg whites mixture into the chocolate and then lastly, fold it with the remaining half of the egg white mixture. Gently fold in almond meal plus the shot of coffee and raspberries. Bake for 30-40 minutes.

Choco Muffins

Ingredients:
½ cup raw pecans, chopped
½ cups almond flour
½ teaspoon ground cinnamon
½ teaspoon salt
1 ½ teaspoon baking soda
1 ½ cups banana
1 egg
1 tablespoon honey
3 tablespoon coconut oil
3 tablespoon coconut cream
½ cup chocolate chips

Procedure:
Preheat the oven to 350°F. In a bowl, place chopped raw pecans, almond flour, ground cinnamon, salt and baking soda. Set aside. Put in the blender and whirl bananas, egg, honey, coconut oil and coconut cream. Mix this with the dry ingredients. Fold in the chocolate chips. Place the batter in muffin cups and bake for approximately 15 minutes.

Chocolate with banana

Ingredients:
2 cups almond butter
3 eggs
1 cup honey
1 tablespoon vanilla
½ teaspoon sea salt
1 teaspoon baking soda
½ cup melted dark chocolate
1 ripe banana, mashed
½ cup chocolate chips

Procedure:
Preheat the oven to 325°F. Make a smooth batter by blending almond butter and eggs. Add honey and vanilla. Mix well. Add sea salt, baking soda and slowly add melted dark chocolate. Fold in a very ripe banana and chocolate, mix well. Bake for 30-45 minutes.

Ultimate Brownie

Ingredients:
1 peeled and grated white sweet potato
2 eggs
2 teaspoon vanilla
½ cup honey
½ cup olive oil
1 tablespoon baking powder
½ tablespoon baking soda
1 cup unsweetened cocoa powder
2 tablespoon coconut flour

Procedure:
Preheat the oven to 350°F. Combine in a bowl white sweet potato, eggs, vanilla and honey. Mix well. Add olive oil and baking powder. Mix well again. Lastly, add baking soda, unsweetened cocoa powder and coconut flour. Place in a lightly greased baking pan. Bake for 30-45 minutes. Top with raspberries or chocolate chips or both.

Macaroons

Ingredients:
¾ cup egg whites
3 tablespoon honey
1 tablespoon vanilla
3 cups shredded coconut

Procedure:
Preheat the oven to 350°F. Beat thoroughly egg whites and then add honey and vanilla. Carefully fold in shredded coconut (one cup at a time). Place the mixture on a parchment paper lined baking pan and bake for 15 minutes. Drizzle melted chocolate on top of the macaroons.

Chocolate Cake with Apricots

Ingredients:
3 eggs, separated
½ teaspoon cream of tartar
1 cup chestnut flour
½ cup almond flour
½ cup raw cacao powder
½ cup coconut sugar
¾ cup coconut milk
½ teaspoon baking soda
3 ripe, peeled, diced apricots

Procedure:
Preheat the oven to 350°F. In a bowl, mix egg whites and cream of tartar until stiff peaks form. Set it aside. In another bowl, mix the egg yolks, chestnut flour, almond flour, raw cacao powder, coconut sugar, coconut milk, baking soda. Fold in the egg whites. Fold in ripe, peeled and diced apricots. Pour into a lightly greased pie mold and bake for 30-45 minutes.

These drinks are not just drinks but can also serve as desserts!

1. ***Chocolate Shake it!*** – Place in a blender 6-8 cubes of ice, ½ cup coconut milk, ½ water and 2 tablespoons raw cacao powder and a sweetener of your choice. Blend until the cubes of ice are crushed. It's refreshing and healthy!

2. ***Raspberry Frappe*** – Combine 1 1/2 cup frozen raspberries, 6-7 pieces mint leaves, 1 teaspoon maple syrup and 1/2 cup orange juice. Blend until smooth.

3. ***Smoothie Delight-*** Place the following in a high speed blender: 1 cup frozen mixed berries, 1 ripe banana, 1 cup fresh squeezed orange juice, ½ cup unsweetened almond milk, 1 teaspoon honey. Whirl until smooth.

4. ***Berry Shake-*** In a blender put: ½ cup milk, ½ cup frozen berries. Sprinkle gelatin and blend until smooth. Add sweetener to the taste.

5. ***Heart to Heart*** – This is very simple but very heart warming. Place sliced red pomegranates on an ice cube tray that is heart-shaped. Add water. Let it freeze. When serving the dessert, place the heart shaped ice into a transparent drink or water.

6. ***Paleo Strawberry and Coconut Smoothie*** – Put in a blender the following, 3 strawberries, 1 cup coconut milk, 1

teaspoon honey. Whirl until it is smooth and creamy. Place in the refrigerator or serve as is.

7. ***Coffee Frappe***–Place in a blender and mix thoroughly the following: ¼ cup brewed coffee, ½ teaspoon vanilla, 1 cup coconut milk, 1 teaspoon maple syrup and 1 cup crushed ice. Ready to drink!

8. ***Mango Smoothie*** – Blend all these and serve immediately: 1 mango, ½ lime – just the juice, 1 kiwi fruit and 1 cup coconut milk. That's it!

9. ***Salted Caramel Shake***–You will need to blend ½ cup coconut milk, 1 ½ teaspoon cashew butter, 1/3 banana, 2 dried pitter dates, a pinch of sea salt, and 1 teaspoon maple syrup plus a couple of ice.

10. ***Pineapple Colada*** –Place in the blender and whirl the following: 1 cup pineapple juice, 1 cup coconut milk, lime juice, 1 banana and a few ice cubes. Ready to serve!

11. ***Paleo Maple Drink*** – Place 8 ounces water in a glass and stir in 1 tablespoon of maple syrup. Drink warm or with ice.

12. ***3 Fruit Smoothie*** – You will need to blend 1 ½ frozen bananas, 1 cup frozen blueberries and 1 cup frozen strawberries. Add 1 cup coconut milk and 1 cup acai juice plus some ice cubes.

13. ***Watermelon and Lime Combo***- combine 2 cups watermelon, 1 lime (juice only), 1 teaspoon honey and a couple of ice cubes in a blender. Blend until smooth.

14. ***Apple Cinnamon Shake*** - Use the blender to mix the following: 1 cup apple, 1 tablespoon honey, 1 teaspoon cinnamon, ½ teaspoon vanilla and add cashew nuts if you like.

15. ***Banana Drink*** - Place 2 pieces ripe banana, ½ cup coconut milk, 1 tablespoon honey and ½ cup water in a blender. Whirl until smooth and serve with ice.

16. ***Iced Coffee Goodness***– Pour ice over a brewed coffee in a closed container and shake well. Transfer to a glass and serve!

17. ***Fruit Salad Drink*** – Put in a glass 1 thinly sliced strawberry, 5 blueberries, 5 pomegranates and 1 sliced banana. Add ½ cup sweetened coconut milk. Put some ice cubes and serve.

18. ***Banana And Apple Mix*** – Place 1 peeled ripe banana and 1 peeled and diced apple in a blender. Add ½ teaspoon vanilla extract and 1 tablespoon honey plus ½ cup coconut milk. Whirl until smooth.

Let kids have fun making their own desserts. Share the memories as you help your children develop a love for cooking and healthy foods too. Maintain safety at all times please. Adult supervision is important when the chocolate need to be melted. Allow the kids' imagination and creativity to come to life as you let them design their own desserts!

1. ***Chocolate Covered Berries*** – Kids will surely love these! Oh and adults too! Melt a bar of dark chocolate by using a double boiler. The boiling water on the lower boiler and the chocolate on top. When the chocolate is already melted, just dip in a clean berry and that's it.

2. ***Pineapple-Banana Popsicles*** – Allow the kids to pour the following into the blender: one 6-ounce can of pineapple juice, 1 banana, ½ teaspoon of vanilla and 1 can coconut milk. Let the adults blend this until smooth. Pour into the popsicle shells and freeze. Sometimes, you might need to soak your popsicle tray in warm water so that they will come out.

3. ***Luscious Looking Popsicle Strawberry*** - pour 1 cup of coconut milk, 3 strawberries, 1 tablespoon honey into a blender. Let the adults use the blender until it is smooth. Pour into the popsicle shells. Let it freeze.

4. ***Layered Delight*** - Get a container. Fill the bottom with a layer of jelly (ask an adult to make this). Put the sliced

mango on top of the jelly layer. Then follow it up with diced Paleo cake (ask and adult to buy this- they are ready made at your local store). Then place bananas on top and follow it up with 8 ounces coconut cream. Finally, on top, you can garnish with some berries, nuts or more mangoes. Decorate as you wish. Set in the freezer and after 2-3 hours, it's ready to be eaten.

5. ***Chocolate Popsicle*** –Allow an adult to melt the chocolate. Pour it on a kiddie shaped design container then add the popsicle sticks. Place in the refrigerator to set.

6. ***DIY Banana Split***–If you have a homemade strawberry or chocolate ice cream, design it with a banana, chocolate chips and maple syrup.

7. ***Easter Bunny Fruit Platter*** – place on your plate the following: 2 apple slices as the ears of the bunny, blueberries as the eyes, 1 peach sliced in half to serve as the cheeks, and 4 pomegranates lined as a smiling mouth. Eat anytime!

8. ***Chocolate Squares*** – Ask an adult to melt a bar of unsweetened chocolate using a double boiler. Remove from heat. Stir the chocolate while you add ½ teaspoon vanilla. Place in a pan and let it set in the refrigerator for 30-45 minutes. You can cut into squares using a plastic knife or ask an adult to cut them for you. Alternatively, add chopped nuts or dried fruit into the melted chocolate.

9. **Cake Pops**–Cake on a popsicle stick! Ask an adult to do this for you. You can design it later. The adult starts by preheating the pop cake maker. Then melt ½ cup dark chocolate with ½ cup coconut milk. Add 2 beaten eggs. Mix well. Add ½ teaspoon vanilla extract, a pinch of sea salt and ¼ teaspoon baking powder. Pipe your batter into the pop cake maker by placing it in a Ziplock bag with a corner trimmed. Close the lid and cook for 5 minutes. Turn the other side and cook for 2 more minutes. Insert the stick and freeze for 30 minutes.

10. **Pop Cakes with Vanilla Glaze**– After making the cake pops, prepare the vanilla glaze using ½ cup coconut butter, 2 tablespoon honey and ½ teaspoon vanilla in a small glass. Warm this glass with warm water (an adult will do this) and decorate your pop cake with the glaze or you can just dip in your pop cake.

11. **Chocolate Glaze Pop Cake-** Or you may want a chocolate glaze. Ask an adult to melt ½ cup chocolate chips. Then dip or decorate your chocolate glaze. Add maple sugar, if desired.

Chapter 6 – Other Goodies

There are so many things you can try with the Paleo desserts. Here are some more recipes!

Apple Cookies

Ingredients:
1 egg, beaten
1 cup unsweetened almond butter
½ cup honey
1 teaspoon baking soda
½ teaspoon sea salt
½ apple, cored, peeled, diced
1 teaspoon cinnamon
1 teaspoon nutmeg
¼ teaspoon ground cloves
1 teaspoon ginger, grated

Procedure:
Simply combine the following in a bowl: 1 beaten egg, 1 cup unsweetened almond butter, ½ cup honey, 1 teaspoon baking soda and ½ teaspoon sea salt. Mix thoroughly. Add the apple, just half of an apple and diced, 1 teaspoon cinnamon, 1/8 teaspoon nutmeg and ¼ teaspoon ground cloves. Then lastly, the ginger, one teaspoon, grated. Spoon the batter and place into a baking sheet. Try to spread the butter 1-2 inches away from each other. Preheat the oven to 350°F and bake the cookies for 10 minutes. Remove from the oven and let it cool for 10 more minutes. Then it is ready to be served!

Very Nutty Cookies

Ingredients:
2 bananas, smashed
1/3 cup coconut flour
¾ cup almond butter
½ teaspoon baking powder
1 apple, cored, peeled, finely chopped
1/3 cup raw walnuts
1/3 cup coconut milk
1 tablespoon cinnamon

Procedure:
Smashed two bananas and add 1/3 cup coconut flour, ¾ cup almond butter and ½ teaspoon baking powder. Mix well. In a blender, put a finely chopped apple and 1/3 cup raw walnut and blend for 20 seconds. Add this to the banana mixture done earlier plus 1/3 cup coconut milk and 1 tablespoon cinnamon powder. Mix thoroughly. Place onto the baking pan, 1-2 inches apart. Preheat the oven to 350°F. Bake for around 25 minutes. You will have around 20 cookies ready to be served!

Blackberry Cobbler

Ingredients:
3 cups fresh blackberries
Honey
1 ½ cups finely ground almonds
2 tablespoon coconut oil
Cinnamon, to taste

Procedure:
Place 3 cups of fresh blackberries in a pie pan. Drizzle a bit of honey on top of the berries. In a separate bowl, mix 1 ½ cups finely ground almonds and 2 tablespoon coconut oil plus add cinnamon according to your taste preference (maybe a pinch or a teaspoon). Mix well. You would expect the mixture to be thick and clumpy. Crumble this on top of the berries and bake for 35 minutes at 350°F.

Mango Ice Cream – You can use a blender or an ice cream maker here.

Ingredients:
3-5 pieces of mango flesh
½ cup coconut milk
½ teaspoon vanilla

Procedure:
Place 3-5 pieces of mango flesh, half cup coconut milk, ½ teaspoon vanilla. Whirl until smooth and then freeze for an hour.

Truly Almond Cookies

Ingredients:
1 ½ cups almond flour
¼ teaspoon salt
¼ teaspoon baking soda
1/8 teaspoon cinnamon
2 tablespoon coconut oil
1 ¼ teaspoon vanilla
¼ teaspoon almond extract
¼ cup maple syrup

Procedure:
In a bowl, put together 1 ½ cups almond flour, ¼ teaspoon salt, ¼ teaspoons baking soda, and 1/8 teaspoon cinnamon. Mix very well, there should be no lumps. In another bowl, mix 2 tablespoons coconut oil, 1 ¼ teaspoon vanilla, ¼ teaspoon almond extract, and ¼ cup maple syrup. Whisk well. Combine the ingredients of the two bowls and stir well. Roll into a ball and then place on a baking pan lined with parchment paper. Flatten the ball slightly and then place one whole almond on the center. Preheat the oven to 325°F and bake for 15-20 minutes. Allow to cool and then serve with Paleo tea.

Grilled Bananas

Ingredients:
4 bananas, quartered
Cinnamon

Procedure:
Quarter 4 bananas (or depending on the number of your guests) and leave the peel on. Sprinkle cinnamon and then grill the open side first for 2-3 minutes only. Flip on the peel side and wait for 2-3 minutes. Serve hot.

Grilled peaches

Ingredients:
Peaches (1 per person)
Cinnamon
Pumpkin pie spice (optional)

Procedure:
Slice the peaches in half and remove the pit. Sprinkle some cinnamon to add to taste. You could also try pumpkin pie spice. Grill for 3-5 minutes and then turn on the other side. Grill too within 3-5 minutes. You may add homemade whipped cream if you desire.

Vanilla Fruit Dip

Ingredients:
1 teaspoon vanilla extract
1 cup coconut milk
2 ripe bananas
2 teaspoon coconut flour

Procedure:
Put into the blender 1 teaspoon vanilla extract, 1 cup coconut milk, 2 ripe bananas and 2 teaspoons coconut flour. Whirl for 2-3

minutes until smooth. Serve with slices of peaches, strawberries or apples.

Fried Apples Dessert

Ingredients:
2 tablespoon coconut oil
3-4 apples, thinly sliced
¼ cup raisins
½ tablespoon cinnamon
2 tablespoon canned coconut milk

Procedure:
In a pan, heat 2 tablespoons coconut oil over medium heat. Add 3-4 apples, thinly sliced. Add ¼ cup raisins for 2 minutes. Then add ½ tablespoon cinnamon and 2 tablespoons canned coconut milk. Stir well and it's ready to be served!

Coconut Macaroons

Ingredients:
16 ounces unsweetened coconut
¼ teaspoon cream of tartar
6 egg whites
1 teaspoon vanilla extract
1 cup honey

Procedure:
Cook unsweetened coconut (around 16 ounces) until it turns golden brown in color. In a separate bowl, using a mixer with a whisk attachment, beat ¼ teaspoon cream of tartar and 6 egg whites. Mix until hard peaks form and mixture is glossy. Stir in 1 teaspoon vanilla extract, 1 cup honey and the golden brown coconut cooked earlier. Mold the mixture into little balls and place on the baking pan. Preheat oven at 350°F. Bake for 10-12 minutes.

Pancake Special

Ingredients:
4 eggs, beaten
¼ cup coconut flour
¼ teaspoon vanilla
1 pinch nutmeg
1 pinch cinnamon
¼ cup coconut milk

Procedure:
Pour 4 beaten eggs into a bowl. Add ¼ cup coconut flour, ¼ teaspoon vanilla, 1 pinch nutmeg, 1 pinch cinnamon and ¼ cup coconut milk. Cook like the usual pancake by putting oil on a pan and pouring about ¼ cup of batter. Flip to the other side when it turns brown. Serve with honey or strawberry.

Nuts about Coconut

Ingredients:
2 cups coconut milk
1 tablespoon cacao powder
10 dates, seeds removed
2 tablespoon coconut cream

Procedure:
Place the following into a blender: 2 cups coconut milk, 1 tablespoon cacao powder, 10 dates with seeds removed and 2 tablespoon coconut cream. Blend thoroughly. Place into a container lined with parchment paper and freeze. Once it sets, you can slice and serve.

Caramel Topping

Ingredients:
2 tablespoon hulled tahini
1 tablespoon honey
2 tablespoon coconut milk
½ teaspoon vanilla

Procedure:
Put 2 tablespoons of hulled tahini and 1 tablespoon honey and mix with a fork. Add 2 tablespoons of coconut milk and ½ teaspoon of vanilla. Place on top of your ice cream for a more delightful dessert!

Triple Fruit Layer

Ingredients:
3-5 sliced pieces of peaches
Fruit jelly
Coconut cream
1 teaspoon honey
1 mango, sliced

Procedure:
Prepare a container. On the bottom, place 3-5 sliced pieces of peaches. On top of the peaches, layer it up with jelly. Then brush it with a small amount of coconut cream and a teaspoon of honey evenly spread. The next layer is a layer of sliced mangos, followed with coconut cream again. Spread a variety of berries on top. Put in the freezer until it sets.

Partner for Muffins

Ingredients:
5 dates
½ cup water
2 ½ tablespoon coconut flour
1 egg
1 ripe banana, peeled
½ teaspoon baking powder

Procedure:
Heat 5 pieces of dates with a half cup water over low heat until the dates break down. Mash the dates and set aside. Blend by use of food processor 2 ½ tablespoon coconut flour, one egg, 1 ripe and peeled banana and ½ teaspoon baking powder. Combine the dates and this mixture. Cook in the oven for 20 minutes. Place this cooked yummy sweet mixture on top of your muffins.

Cool Ice Cream

Ingredients:
4 bananas, frozen
4 tablespoon coconut milk
1 teaspoon vanilla

Procedure:
Simply blend 4 frozen bananas, 4 tablespoons coconut milk and 1 teaspoon vanilla and place in the freezer for an hour or so.

Paleo Fruit Salad 1

Ingredients:
1 cup kiwi, peeled
1 apple, diced
1 mango, peeled and diced
1 peach, cut in half and pitted
½ cup coconut milk

Procedure:
Place in a big bowl 1 cup peeled kiwi, 1 diced apple, 1 mango, peeled and diced, and 2 pieces peach. Add ½ cup coconut milk. Chill and serve.

Paleo Fruit Salad 2

Ingredients:
2 ripe bananas
1 coconut, shredded flesh

Procedure:
Another combination that will suit the palate is this: add 2 pieces ripe bananas and 1 shredded coconut flesh to the Paleo Fruit Salad 1

Fruits and Nuts

Ingredients:
3 dates, pitted
2 ripe bananas
½ cup almond butter
½ teaspoon nutmeg
¼ teaspoon ground cloves
½ teaspoon baking soda
½ cup pecans, crushed
½ teaspoon lemon extract

Procedure:
Preheat oven to 350°F. Blend 3 pitted dates, 2 ripe bananas, ½ cup almond butter, ½ teaspoon nutmeg, ¼ teaspoon ground cloves, ½ teaspoon baking soda, ½ cup crushed pecans and ½ teaspoon lemon extract. Whirl until smooth. Scoop the batter and place on the baking pan. Bake for 10-15 minutes. Allow to cool.

Orange Cake Delight

Ingredients:
2 oranges, peeled
1 banana, peeled
3 eggs
4 tablespoon coconut sugar
2 cups almond meal
1 teaspoon baking powder

Procedure:
Preheat oven to 350°F. Blend 2 peeled oranges and 1 banana. Set aside. Beat 3 eggs and add 4 tablespoon coconut sugar. Mix well. Add to this 2 cups of almond meal, orange and banana mix, and 1 teaspoon baking powder. Pour to the baking tin. Bake for one hour. Allow to cool.

Sweet Bananas

Ingredients:
½ cup water
2 bananas, sliced
½ teaspoon vanilla extract
1 tablespoon maple syrup
½ cup cold coconut milk

Procedure:
In a pan, place the following over medium heat. ½ cup water, 2 piece sliced ripe bananas, ½ teaspoon vanilla extract and 1 tablespoon maple syrup. Cook until it thickens. Let it cool for 10 minutes. Pour ½ cup cold coconut milk and then serve.

Paleo Refrigerator Cake

This recipe is very similar to the usual refrigerator cake but with a touch of the Paleo ingredients.

Ingredients:
Paleo cake
1 mango, sliced
Coconut cream

Procedure:
Place a layer of homemade Paleo sponge cake (or you can buy this) onto the bottom of a container. Next, make a layer of sliced mango. Pour coconut cream on top and spread evenly. Layer again with the remaining sponge cake. On top, you can decorate your refrigerator cake with different berries.

Fudgy Espresso Brownie

Ingredients:
1 cup cocoa or cacao powder
5 walnut pieces
1 cup strong expresso

Procedure:
Blend 1 cup of cocoa powder and 5 pieces of walnuts. Add a cup of strong espresso. Whirl in a blender. After they are totally blended, roll these into small balls. Coffee and brownie all in one!

Upside Down Banana Cake

Ingredients:
2 tablespoon coconut butter, melted
2 tablespoon coconut sugar
1 teaspoon cinnamon
1 banana, sliced
2 eggs
1/3 maple syrup
¼ cup unsweetened coconut milk
1 teaspoon vanilla extract
½ teaspoon baking soda
1 teaspoon apple cider vinegar
1 small banana, mashed
1/3 cup coconut flour

Procedure:
Preheat oven to 350°F. Put 2 tablespoon melted butter on the baking pan. Sprinkle 2 tablespoon coconut sugar evenly on top of the melted butter. Then sprinkle 1 teaspoon cinnamon. Layer one sliced banana next. In a bowl, mix 2 eggs, 1/3 maple syrup, ¼ cup unsweetened coconut milk, 1 teaspoon vanilla extract, ½ teaspoon baking soda, 1 teaspoon apple cider vinegar and 1 small mashed banana. Mix well. Add 1/3 cup coconut flour. There should be no lumps. Place on the pan and bake for approximately 25 minutes. Slice and serve upside down.

Apple Cinnamon Cake

Ingredients:
½ cup almond flour
¼ cup arrowroot starch
1/3 cup coconut sugar
2 tablespoon almond
1 tablespoon cinnamon
1 teaspoon baking powder
¼ teaspoon salt
1 tablespoon almond or coconut butter
2 eggs, beaten
½ cup coconut milk
1 teaspoon vanilla
1 cup apple, grated

Procedure:
Place in a food processor the following dry ingredients: ½ cup almond flour, ¼ cup arrowroot starch, 1/3 cup coconut sugar, 2 tablespoons flour, 1 tablespoon cinnamon, 1 teaspoon baking powder and ¼ teaspoon salt. Whirl for a few times. Add 1 tablespoon butter and whirl. In a bowl, mix 2 beaten eggs, ½ cup coconut milk, 1 teaspoon vanilla. Add 1 cup grated apple and stir. Add to the food processor. Pour the mixture into the baking pan and bake for 30 minutes. Serve as it is or add a topping like the next recipe.

Apple Cinnamon Cake with Walnut Topping

Ingredients:
1 ½ cups walnuts
½ cup coconut flour
4 tablespoon coconut butter
2 tablespoon coconut sugar
Pinch of salt
1 tablespoon cinnamon

Procedure:
Make a topping by mixing the following ingredients: 1 ½ cups walnuts, ½ cup flour, 4 tablespoons melted butter, 2 tablespoon coconut sugar, a pinch of salt and 1 tablespoon cinnamon. Whirl in the food processor and then sprinkle on top of your apple cinnamon cake.

Simply Orange Cake

Ingredients:
2 oranges
6 eggs, beaten
10.5 ounces almond meal
3.5 ounces coconut syrup
1 teaspoon baking soda

Procedure:
Preheat the oven to 325°F. Boil 2 oranges in a saucepan for about 2 hours. Blend thoroughly the oranges and 6 beaten eggs in a processor. Add 10.5 ounces almond meal, 3.5 ounces coconut syrup and 1 teaspoon baking soda. Mix well and then place batter on the baking pan and bake for 45 minutes.

Peanut Butter Delight

Ingredients:
5 tablespoon sunflower seed butter
1 tablespoon honey
1 tablespoon coconut oil
1 tablespoon flaxseed meal
1 tablespoon vanilla
¾ cup almond flour
Pinch of salt
¼ cup chocolate chips
1 tablespoon cacao butter
Chopped almonds

Procedure:
In a large bowl, mix with your gloved hand the following ingredients: 5 tablespoons sunflower seed butter, 1 tablespoon each of honey, coconut oil, and flaxseed meal, 2 tablespoon vanilla, ¾ cup almond flour and a pinch of salt. Roll the dough into a ball and refrigerate for 30 minutes. Melt ¼ cup chocolate chips and 1 tablespoon cacao butter. Dip the balls into this and top with chopped almonds. Refrigerate until firm and then serve!

Raw Brownie Bites

Ingredients:
1½ cups walnuts
Pinch of salt
1cup pitted dates
1 teaspoon vanilla
1/3 cup unsweetened cocoa powder

Procedure:
Add walnuts and salt to a blender or food processor. Mix until the walnuts are finely ground. Add the dates, vanilla, and cocoa powder to the blender. Mix well until everything is combined. With the blender still running, add a couple drops of water at a time to make the mixture stick together. Using a spatula, transfer the mixture into a bowl. Using your hands, form small round balls, rolling in your palm. Store in an airtight container in the refrigerator for up to a week.

Paleo Chocolate Cupcakes

Ingredients:
4 eggs
1/2 cup honey
1/3 cup coconut flour
1/4 cup cacao powder
1/2 teaspoon baking soda
1/4 cup coconut oil (melted in microwave)
1/4 cup cacao butter (melted in microwave)

For topping:
1 can coconut cream (chilled in fridge overnight)
Honey (optional)
1/4 cup jam or coulis (See my easy jam recipe here.)
Cacao nibs to decorate.

Procedure:
Heat the oven to 170° Celsius (338° F). Grease 10 muffin pans with coconut oil. Beat eggs and honey with electric beaters. Add coconut flour, baking soda and cacao powder. Beat well. Add melted coconut oil, cacao butter and mix. Spoon mixture into 10 greased muffin pans. Bake for 12-15 minutes until risen and top springs back.

Cool in pans. Beat the solid coconut cream with electric beaters until creamy. Add honey to taste if you wish. Pipe coconut cream onto top of cakes. Drizzle with jam or coulis.

Chocolate "Peanut Butter" Ice Cream with Chocolate Shell

Ingredients:
For the ice cream
2 (14 ounce) cans coconut milk
3 tablespoons unsweetened cocoa powder
⅓ cup raw honey
1 teaspoon instant coffee (I used ground coffee)
⅛ teaspoon cinnamon
Pinch of salt
¼ cup sunflower seed butter (or other nut butter)

For the chocolate shell
¼ cup coconut oil, melted
1 tablespoon unsweetened cocoa powder
1 tablespoon sunbutter (or other nut butter)
2 tablespoons raw honey
½ teaspoon vanilla extract
Pinch of salt

Procedure:
Place a saucepan over medium heat and add all ice cream ingredients to it, except for the sunflower seed butter. Stir until cocoa powder is completely broken down and ingredients are smooth. Place saucepan in the freezer until cool. Mine took about an hour. Pour ice cream ingredients in your ice cream maker and turn on. When ice cream is almost done mixing, pour in the sunflower seed butter directly into the ice cream maker to churn with your chocolate ice cream. While ice cream is churning, place the chocolate shell ingredients in a bowl and in the microwave for about 30 seconds until everything is mixed. Whisk together until smooth. When ice cream is done churning, place in bowl and bowl chocolate shell on top!

Strawberries& Cream Ice Cream with Almond Butter Crisp

Ingredients:
For the Ice Cream:
1 can full fat coconut milk
3 tablespoon honey
2 tablespoon vanilla
1 cup fresh strawberries, cut into fourths
For the crisp:
1/3 cup almond flour
3 tablespoon sunflower seed butter (or almond butter)
1/2 teaspoon vanilla
1 tablespoon honey
salt to taste

Procedure:

For the ice cream:

Combine coconut milk, honey, and vanilla together in a small saucepan over medium heat and stir until ingredients are well combined (just a few minutes). Transfer milk mixture to a small bowl and place in the freezer for two hours. Next, add strawberries to a small saucepan and bring to a low boil. Turn heat to medium-low and allow to cook until they start breaking down into a sauce-like mixture, leaving small chunks. Place strawberries in refrigerator while the ice cream hardens.

For the crisp:

Combine all ingredients and mix until you get a "crumble' consistency. Place crisp in refrigerator until ready to use. After two hours, place milk mixture into your ice cream maker along with the strawberries and use as directed. When ice cream is ready, scoop and serve with crisp sprinkled on top.

Paleo White Chocolate

Ingredients:
1/4 cup of raw cacao butter, melted
1 teaspoon maple sugar
1 teaspoon of vanilla powder
2 ounces coconut milk powder
Tiny pinch of salt
1 teaspoon cacao nibs (optional for inside your chocolates)

Procedure:
Melt your raw cocoa butter in a glass bowl over a double boiler on your stove set to low (raw cocoa melts at 93 degrees, don't burn it). Once melted, transfer to another bowl and add the remaining ingredients. Whisk well ensuring there are no lumps left and everything is incorporated. Transfer to a blender or a food processor and run it to get it as smooth as possible. Pour into your chocolate molds or silicon cups and place in the freezer for at least an hour. Remove and serve or chop them up and add them to chocolate chip cookies or muffins

Paleo Chocolate Chip Pizookie

Ingredients:
2 cups sifted blanched almond flour
1/2 teaspoon baking soda
1/4 teaspoon sea salt
1 cup Enjoy Life Mini Chocolate Chips (soy free, dairy free)
1 organic cage-free egg
1/3 cup raw honey (melted)
1/4 cup coconut oil (melted)
1/2 teaspoon vanilla Extract

Procedure:
Preheat oven to 350 °F. Grease mini 6″ cast iron skillets. In a large bowl, mix together the almond flour, baking soda, and salt with a fork. Add the chocolate chips to the dry mixture and combine. In a small separate bowl, mix the wet ingredients together, honey, coconut oil, vanilla extract, and egg. You may need to heat the honey and coconut oil in order to liquefy them, remember to heat before you add the egg. Stir the wet ingredients into the dry until evenly mixed. Let the dough chill in the fridge for at least 30 minutes. Then fill both skillets evenly with dough. Bake for 30-35 minutes or until a toothpick comes out clean. Garnish with coconut milk ice cream and enjoy!

Blueberry Mango Muffins

Ingredients:
3 eggs
3 tablespoon honey
2 tablespoon coconut oil, melted
2 tablespoon coconut milk
1/4 teaspoon salt
1/4 teaspoon vanilla
1/4 teaspoon baking powder
1/4 cup coconut flour
1/2 cup diced mango
1/2 cup blueberries

Procedure:
Preheat oven to 400°F. Mix together your eggs, honey, coconut oil, coconut milk, salt and vanilla. Sift together your baking powder and coconut flour and then combine with your wet ingredients. Mix your batter well and then fold in your diced mango and blueberries. If not, divide your batter into 9 muffin tins and bake for 20 minutes or until done.

Dark Chocolate Fudge Pops

Ingredients:
1¼ cups coconut milk
2 egg yolks
½ cup maple syrup or honey
Dash of sea salt
1½ teaspoons unflavored gelatin
1 teaspoon vanilla extract
2 ounces unsweetened chocolate, roughly chopped

Procedure:
Soften the gelatin by placing it in a small bowl with the vanilla extract. Warm the coconut milk over medium-high heat for 6-7 minutes, being careful not to let it boil. Whisk the egg yolks, maple syrup, and salt in a small bowl. Slowly pour the hot coconut milk into the egg mixture, whisking continuously to temper the eggs. Pour the entire liquid mixture back into the pan, and continue cooking over medium high heat for 6-8 minutes while stirring constantly. You don't want this mixture to boil and it should be thick enough to coat the back of a spoon. Pour the softened gelatin and vanilla into the pan and whisk vigorously until the gelatin has completely dissolved, about 2 minutes. Remove from heat, and pour the mixture into a glass bowl. *If you notice a few small lumps, pass it through a mesh strainer prior to pouring it into the bowl.* Stir in the chopped chocolate until it is incorporated and smooth, then let the pudding cool for 20 minutes at room temperature. Pour the pudding into popsicle molds and freeze for at least 6 hours until solid.

Sweet Spinach Pie with Basic Paleo Almond Crust

Ingredients:
For the pie crust:
1 cup ground almonds (almond flour)
1 tablespoon coconut flour
1 tablespoon coconut oil
1 egg
Pinch of sea salt

For the spinach filling:
300g fresh spinach leaves (1 cup cooked)
4 eggs, separated
1 cup ground almonds (almond flour)
2 tablespoons coconut flour
1 cup coconut sugar
1 teaspoon rosewater
Pinch of sea salt

Procedure:
For the crust:
In a mixing bowl, knead all the ingredients together until a dough is formed. With your hands, press the dough into a pie plate, bottom and sides (I used a 6-inch round plate). Set aside.

For the spinach filling:
In a medium-sized pot, place the spinach and about 1 cup of water. At medium heat, bring to a boil, and cook about 5 minutes. Reduce the heat to low and cook an additional 5 minutes. Turn heat off and allow to cool in the pot with water. Once the spinach is cool, drain into a colander and press the spinach to remove all of the water. I pressed it with the back of a spoon. Put the spinach, egg yolks, rosewater and sea salt into a food processor. Pulse until a puree is formed, about 1 minute. Add the almond four, coconut flour and sugar and pulse again until everything is well incorporated. Pour the dough into a mixing bowl. Beat the egg whites until stiff peaks form. Fold the egg whites into the spinach

mixture. Mix well until no white is visible. Pour the spinach filling into the pie crust. Bake at 180°C (350°F) for 35-45 minutes, or until an inserted toothpick comes out dry.

Grilled Peaches with Coconut Cream

Ingredients:
3 medium ripe peaches, cut in half with pit removed
1 teaspoon vanilla
1 can coconut milk, refrigerated
1/4 cup chopped walnuts
Cinnamon (to taste)

Procedure:
Place peaches on the grill with the cut side down first. Grill on medium-low heat until soft, about 3-5 minutes on each side. Scoop cream off the top of the can of chilled coconut milk. Whip together coconut cream and vanilla with handheld mixer. Drizzle over each peach. Top with cinnamon and chopped walnuts to garnish.

No-Bake Mini Pumpkin Bites

Ingredients:

FOR CRUST:
1 cup hazelnuts
1/2 cup raw pumpkin seeds
8 date, pitted
1 tablespoon coconut oil
1 tablespoon REAL maple syrup or raw honey
2 pinches of Celtic sea salt

FOR FILLING:
1 cup cooked pumpkin puree
1/2 cup coconut butter
2 tablespoon coconut oil
3 tablespoon REAL maple syrup or raw honey
1/2 teaspoon vanilla extract
1/4 teaspoon cinnamon powder
1/4 teaspoon ginger powder
1/8 teaspoon allspice
1/8 teaspoon clove powder

FOR CHOCOLATE DRIZZLE:
2 tablespoons coconut butter
2 tablespoons coconut oil
2 tablespoons raw cacao
3 tablespoons REAL maple syrup or raw honey
Pinch or 2 of salt

Procedure:
To make the crust: Line mini muffin tins with unbleached mini paper liners. Process all crust ingredients in a food processor until well combined and resembles a coarse flour. Spoon 1 and 1/2 teaspoon of mixture into each of the 24 mini cups. Use your thumb to press down mixture firmly to create a solid bottom layer for these cute little yummies. Place in freezer to harden.

To make filling: Melt coconut butter and coconut oil in a double boiler. Remove from heat and add rest of filling ingredients. Go ahead and mix it up real good here until creamy smooth. Remove crusts from freezer and spoon about 3/4 TBS of filling over your prepared crusts. Return to freezer to harden, at least 2 hours.

To make chocolate drizzle: Once mini bites have hardened, gently melt coconut butter and coconut oil in a double boiler. Remove from heat and add rest of drizzle ingredients. Allow to cool slightly to thicken. Pour into small plastic bag, cut a TINY hole in the corner, and drizzle over treats in any fashion that you want.

Now it's time to enjoy these amazing delights. Store leftovers in freezer as they are best cold.

Chocolate Hazelnut Cups

Makes about 16-18 cups.

Ingredients:
Two 10 ounce bags of chopped hazelnuts (or almonds, or any nut)
One 10 ounce bag of dark chocolate chips
Two tablespoons of coconut oil--one for the chocolate and one for the nuts

Procedure:
Melt the chocolate over low heat, stirring in a tablespoon of coconut oil once the chips are melted. While your chocolate is melting, add the hazelnuts to a food processor and blend. That's seriously it. It takes a few minutes, but you'll have hazelnut butter before you know it. Throw in a tablespoon of coconut oil for good measure. Spoon some melted chocolate into the bottoms of your candy molds. Add a bit of hazelnut butter. Top it with another spoonful of chocolate. Stick them in the freezer until they've hardened and pop them out. Store them in the refrigerator. Share them with someone you really like.

Cherry Vanilla Ice Crème

Ingredients:

2 14oz. cans Coconut Milk (Full Fat)
1 cup raw honey
1 ½ teaspoon vanilla extract
2 cup fresh Rainier cherries, pitted and diced

Procedure:
In a large bowl, combine coconut milk, honey, and vanilla and stir well. Chill for 1-2 hours. Transfer to ice-cream maker and process according to manufacturer directions. Add diced cherries to the mixture during the last 5-10 minutes of processing.

Apple Pie Caveman Bars

Ingredients:
2 cups dates, pitted
1/2 cup raw macadamia nuts
1/2 cup dried apples
1/4 cup raw almonds
2 tablespoon coconut oil, melted
2 tablespoon cinnamon

Procedure:
Place your dates, macadamia nuts, apples, and almonds in a food processor or really strong blender. Pulse until your dates, macadamia nuts, and almonds are in small chunks and transfer to a mixing bowl. Add in all remaining ingredients. Using your hands mix well to ensure an even coating of everything. Once mixed, using parchment paper, flatten out your mixture to the size of bars you want or you can use individual ziploc bags and form them inside the bag. Place in refrigerator and let cool, then enjoy

Paleo Blueberry and Blackberry Crumble

Ingredients:
2 cups fresh blueberries
2 cups fresh blackberries
Juice from a fresh lemon
1 cup almond flour
¼ cup chopped walnuts
4 pitted dried dates
½ teaspoon cinnamon
¼ teaspoon salt
¼ cup coconut oil, melted
¼ cup sliced almonds

Procedure:
Preheat oven to 350°F. Place the berries in a 9 inch x 9 inch baking dish, and squeeze juice from half of the lemon over and mix. Press the fruit gently into place and rest at room temperature. In a food processor, combine the almond flour, dates, walnuts, cinnamon, and salt. Pulse until combined. Add in the coconut oil and process on high for 5-10 seconds, or until thoroughly combined. Pour topping into a bowl and mix in the sliced almonds. Sprinkle topping over the berries and lightly press into the fruit with a spoon. Bake for 30-40 minutes, until browned.

German Apple Pancake

Ingredients:
6 eggs
1 cup almond milk
3 tablespoon coconut oil, melted
2 teaspoon vanilla
2 teaspoon pure maple syrup
1/4 cup coconut flour
1/2 teaspoon baking soda
1/8 teaspoon nutmeg
2 apples, cored and diced
2 tablespoon coconut oil
2 tablespoon raw organic honey
1 teaspoon cinnamon
1 teaspoon nutmeg
juice of 1/2 lemon
handful of crushed pecans

Procedure:
Preheat Oven to 425°F. In a large bowl, whisk eggs, almond milk, coconut oil, vanilla, and maple syrup. In a small bowl, stir coconut flour, nutmeg, and baking soda. Mix dry ingredients into wet ingredients and beat well to combine, set aside while you prepare the apples. In a small frying pan, heat 2 tablespoon coconut oil and raw organic honey. Stir in cinnamon and nutmeg and juice of 1/2 Lemon and cook for 1 minute. Add in your apples and sauté until all your apples are nicely coated. Evenly divide your apple mixture between 8 ramekins greased with coconut oil and then evenly divide your egg mixture on top of the apples between the 8 Ramekins. Place your Ramekins on a baking sheet and bake for 20 minutes at 425 and then reduce heat to 375°F and cook for an additional 20 minutes. Sprinkle with pecans when removed from the oven.

Paleo Chocolate Coffee Coconut Truffle Desserts

Ingredients:
1/2 cup coconut butter
3 tablespoons 100% cocoa powder
1 tablespoon ground coffee
1 tablespoon unsweetened coconut flakes
1/2 teaspoon raw honey
1 tablespoon coconut oil

Procedure:
Melt the coconut butter (in a microwave) so that it can be mixed with a fork. Mix in all the ingredients (except the coconut oil) and mix well with a fork. Take an ice-cube tray and pour approximately 1/4 teaspoon of coconut oil into 6-7 of the cups. Spoon the mixture into each cup of the ice-cube tray and gently pat them flat with a fork. Freeze for 4-5 hours. Defrost at room temperature for 15-20 minutes before serving.

Fudgy Espresso Brownies

Ingredients:
For the Brownie
6 tablespoons non-dairy butter
6 ounces chocolate
2 tablespoons coconut flour
¼ cup plus 2 tablespoons tapioca flour
1 cup Sucanat or palm sugar
¼ cup strong hot coffee
¼ cup unsweetened cocoa powder
2 eggs
½ teaspoon baking soda
¼ teaspoon salt
Extra butter for pan greasing

For the Mocha Frosting
¼ cup non-dairy butter, melted
¼ cup non-dairy butter, softened
¼ cup strong hot coffee
¾ cup Sucanat or palm sugar

Procedure:
For the Brownie
Preheat the oven to 350°F. Grease an 8x8 baking pan and line with parchment paper. Ensure eggs are at room temperature. You may run them under warm water for about 10 seconds while shelled. Gently melt the semisweet chocolate and butter in a double boiler. You may use the microwave at 50% heat at 30 second intervals with intermittent stirring. Stir in the coffee and unsweetened cocoa powder. Measure the sugar and coconut flour and add to a food processor. Give a few pulses to make a superfine texture. Sift together the superfine coconut flour, sugar, tapioca flour, baking soda, and salt. Beat the eggs and add the dry ingredients. Beat until combined. Add the rest of the wet ingredients and beat until incorporated. Pour the batter into the lined 8x8 pan. Bake for 25-30 minutes at 350F until

a toothpick inserted into the center of the batter comes out clean. When done, remove from the oven and let cool in the pan for at least 15 minutes.

For the Mocha Frosting

Measure the sugar and add to the food processor. Give a few pulses to make a superfine texture. Gently heat the sugar with the ¼ cup of melted butter and coffee until dissolved or mostly dissolved. Refrigerate the mixture for a few hours. It will look terrible at this stage, but don't despair. It is beneficial, but not necessary, to mix every now and then while cooling. When the mixture is cold enough, beat in the softened butter 1 tablespoons at a time on high speed. I find the hand mixer best for this task.

Harvest Pumpkin Custard

Ingredients:
Pumpkin Mix:
1 can pumpkin puree
1 cup coconut cream
3/4 cup raw honey
1 teaspoon pumpkin pie spice
1/4 teaspoon salt

Coconut Whipped Cream:
1 can coconut milk, full fat
1/4 teaspoon vanilla (optional)
1/4 teaspoon cinnamon (optional)

Crumble Mixture:
3/4 cup hazelnut flour
2 teaspoon cinnamon
2 tablespoon coconut sugar

Procedure:

Pumpkin Mix:
In a large metal bowl, combine the pumpkin puree, coconut cream, raw honey, pumpkin pie spice, and salt. Mix until thoroughly combined.

Coconut Whipped Cream:
To make the coconut whipped cream: do not open the can of coconut milk. Place in the refrigerator for at least 2 hours (ideally overnight). Open the can of coconut milk and scoop out thickened coconut cream on top into a bowl. If preferred, you can drink the coconut water or save it for a smoothie. Optional: add cinnamon and vanilla. Finally, whip the coconut cream with a whisk or electric beater until it begins to thicken.

Crumble Mixture:
In another small bowl, combine the hazelnut flour, the cinnamon, and the coconut sugar. Mixed until combined.

In a tall class, mason jars or a large glass dish, alternate the layers of pumpkin mix, coconut cream, and the crumble mixture, ending with the crumble mixture on top. You can choose to in one round of layers or multiple layers.

Choco-Coconut Drops

Ingredients:
3 tablespoon coconut oil
1/2 cup dark chocolate chips
1/4 cup unsweetened cocoa powder
2 tablespoon raw honey
1/4 cup almond butter
1 cup coconut flakes, unsweetened

Procedure:
In a microwave safe bowl, add the coconut oil and chocolate chips. In small increments of time so that the chocolate doesn't burn, cook the mixture at 30 second intervals until the chis are melted. Make sure to stir between each of the 30 second intervals. You can even turn down you power level to further ensure no burning. Once mixture is melted, stir in the cocoa powder, honey, and almond butter. Mix until smooth. Then add the coconut and stir until coated. Drop the batter in scoops on a parchment paper lined baking sheet. Refrigerate the cookies until they are firm. Store leftover in the fridge.

Pecan Caramel Cookie Bark

Ingredients
For the caramel sauce:
1 cup full fat coconut milk
1 cup maple sugar
1 teaspoon vanilla extract
1/4 teaspoon salt

For the bark:
1/3 cup toasted pecans
1 cup mini chocolate chips, melted + extra for garnishing
7-8 gluten free pecan cookies

Procedure:
Make caramel sauce:
Combine all the ingredients in a small saucepan. Place the saucepan over medium heat and stir until completely combined. Once combined, bring to a boil for 12 minutes, ensuring the mixture doesn't boil over. After 12 minutes, lower the heat to a simmer for an additional 5 minutes, or until the caramel lightly coats the back of a spoon. Remove from the heat and let the mixture cool for 5 minutes.

Preheat the oven to 350F. Place the pecans on a baking sheet and roast in over for 10 minutes or until dark and fragrant. Keep an eye on them so they don't burn. As the pecans are roasting, melt the chocolate in a double boiler or in the microwave. Be careful not to burn. Once the chocolate is melted, pour the chocolate on a parchment paper lined baking sheet and spread evenly. Add the cookies and toasted pecans to the melted chocolate. The next step is to use a spoon to spread the caramel throughout the chocolate. Finally, sprinkle the chocolate chips on top. Place the prepared chocolate in the freezer for about 30 minutes to harden. Remove from freezer and break into pieces.

Cookie Dough Bites

Ingredients:
½ cup softened coconut oil
½ cup maple sugar
1 teaspoon vanilla extract
¾ cup cassava flour
pinch of salt
½ cup mini chocolate chips
2 cups mini chocolate chips (or whatever chocolate you prefer), melted

Procedure:
Cream together the coconut oil, sugar and vanilla extract with a hand mixer. Slowly add the cassava flour while the mixer is running until all the flour is combined. Fold in the salt and chocolate chips. Using a spoon or cookie scoop, shape the dough into 12-14 balls. Place the balls in the fridge for 10-15 minutes in order   to   harden.

Melt the chocolate in a microwave or double boiler, being careful not to burn. Using a fork, dip each cookie dough ball into the chocolate and coat all sides. Places the balls in the fridge to harden for about 10 minutes.

Bring the balls to room temperature before serving. Serve with a toothpick.

Strawberry Dark Chocolate Chunk Cookies

Ingredients:
1 cup raw almond butter
1 cup maple sugar
1 egg
1 tablespoon tapioca flour
1 tablespoons coconut flour
1 teaspoon baking soda
1 teaspoon vanilla extract
pinch of salt
3 ounce chocolate bar, roughly chopped
1/3 cup dried strawberries

Procedure:
Preheat oven to 350F and line a baking sheet with parchment paper. In a large mixing bowl, stir together the almond butter and maple sugar. Then add beaten egg. After mixture is combined, add the tapioca and coconut flour, baking soda, vanilla, salt and chocolate chunks. Mix to thoroughly combine.

Using a cookie scoop or spoon, create about 2 tablespoons of dough into a ball. Place on baking sheet. Press a dried strawberry or two into each cookie. Place baking sheet in oven and bake for 10 minutes. Remove from oven and let cool for 10 minutes. If you try to transfer to cooling rack too soon, they will come apart.

Chocolate Truffles

Ingredients:
10 ounces dark chocolate, 70% cacao content or higher
3 tablespoons coconut oil
1 cup full-fat coconut milk
1 teaspoon vanilla extract
½ cup finely shredded unsweetened coconut and/or ½ cup unsweetened cocoa

Procedure:
Place the shredded chocolate and coconut oil in a medium bowl. Set aside for later. In a small saucepan over medium heat, heat the coconut milk until simmering. Once the milk has reached its temperature, pour over the chocolate and coconut mixture. Stir gently with a spatula or spoon to combine. Don't mix too quickly in order to protect the chocolate from becoming grainy. Add the vanilla and stir to combine. Transfer the mixture to a sealed container and chill until solid (at least 4 hours).

Lightly toast the shredded coconut on a parchment-lined baking tray at 300°F oven for 3 to 5 minutes or until golden brown. Move the flakes to a bowl in order to allow them to cool.

Once the chocolate mixture has chilled in the fridge, scoop out 36 balls of chocolate. Roll each ball between your palms to form a smooth ball. Coat the truffle with the toasted coconut. Alternatively, you can use sifted cocoa powder.

No-Bake Pumpkin Bars

Ingredients:
10 pitted Medjool dates
1 cup almonds
1 1/2 tablespoons dark unsweetened cocoa powder
2 teaspoons cinnamon, divided
5 oz. unsweetened coconut flakes, plus more for garnish
1 tablespoon coconut oil, melted
1/2 teaspoon vanilla extract
Pinch of salt
1/3 cup pumpkin puree
1/2 banana
2 tablespoon honey

Procedure:
Cover dates with water in a bowl. Allow to soak for 20-30 minutes to allow for softening. In the meantime, line a 9x5-inch loaf pan with wax paper. In a food processor, place the almonds and pulse to finely chop. Add the soaked dates (drain soaking water), cocoa powder, and 1 teaspoon of cinnamon. Blend the ingredients and the processor until rough dough starts to form. Transfer the dough to the loaf pan and flatten evenly with a spatula. Place the coconut flakes, coconut oil, salt and vanilla in the food processor and mix for at least 1 minute until a paste starts to form. Add this mixture to the loaf pan, spreading evenly over the almond mixture base. Add to the food processor, the pumpkin puree, banana, honey and remaining teaspoon of cinnamon. Blend until smooth. Spread this mixture evenly over the coconut mixture in the loaf pan. Sprinkle with coconut flakes if preferred. Place in freezer for 1 hour. Cut into squares before serving.

Chocolate Mug Cake
1 serving

Ingredients:
1 heaping tablespoon almond flour
1 heaping tablespoon unsweetened cocoa powder
1 tablespoon unsweetened vanilla almond milk
½ tablespoon honey
1 egg
1 teaspoon vanilla extract

Procedure:
In a mug, mix together all the ingredients. Microwave for 1 to 1.5 minutes.

Conclusion

Thank you again for this book!

I hope this book was able to help you to enjoy your sweets without the guilt and without compromise to your health!

The next step is to go out and start buying those prehistoric ingredients at your local grocery stores. Have fun exploring your creativity and finding new ways to enjoy sweets!

In addition, please remember to check out our Facebook page in order to find other resources and upcoming promotions:

https://www.facebook.com/joypublishing

With sincere thanks,

Emma Rose

Preview Of "Paleo Free Diet Guide for Beginners: Over 50 Paleo Free Diet Recipes for Fast Weight Loss and Optimal Health"

Introduction

I want to thank you and congratulate you for purchasing this book!

This book contains everything you might need to know when it comes to getting started with the Paleo Free Diet. It is provided in an easily digestible format that allows you to better absorb the information. There are no complicated explanations about how it works! You'll be given what you need straight up so you won't have to waste time trying to understand exactly what the diet is. Whether it's for your overall good health or to lose a few pounds, Paleo can certainly help you with it. To help you get started, we'll do the same and start you off with 50 of the best Paleo recipes that you can slowly but surely shift your everyday menu to.

It's never easy changing a diet. I often fall into self-pity when I can no longer have the foods I enjoy. Either I feel sorry for myself or I get rebellious and binge and anything and everything. I always knew the value of eating healthy. I could just never bring myself to do it. It wasn't until I had a miscarriage that I got serious about my health. I have made drastic changes that others just don't understand. But the payoff is the weight I've lost and the better health I'm experiencing.

My hope for you is not to be on another "diet." This isn't a restriction diet like Atkins. The goal is to have a lifestyle change. Lifestyle changes are more sustainable and maintain weight loss long term compared to restriction diets. The change is hard to start but worth it when you commit. The trick is to get the momentum to start.

Thanks again for purchasing this book. I hope you enjoy reading it and eating the recipes from it!

With gratitude,

Emma Rose

Chapter 1 – What Is the Paleo Free Diet?

The Paleo Free Diet is known by many names such as the cavemen diet, stone age diet and hunter-gatherer diet, to name a few. The concept behind this diet follows that of the Paleolithic era before the development of agriculture. Essentially, you consume the same foods that the cavemen used to eat. The focus is on eating food closest to its natural, unprocessed state. The cavemen would gather their food from any source available whether it was wild animals, berries, vegetables, or fruits. As a result, they were strong, fit, and healthy for thousands of years.

This type of diet is still very young, less than fifty years only, but more in depth researches and studies are being conducted to increase the information and knowledge on this diet. The results of previous studies conducted on the Paleo Free Diet reveal the improvement of health to the people involved. This is attributed to the fact that no processed foods and additives are included. The Paleo Free Diet is a diet that works with our genetics – before machinery and processing got involved. Foods that were not available during the Paleolithic time such as dairy products, salt, sugar and grains are not included in the preparation of the Paleo Free Diet.

The modern diet predominately consumed in the Western world is full of refined foods, trans fats, salt and sugar. These ingredients are known to indirectly cause diseases such as hypertension, diabetes, strokes, obesity and other heart problems. The list goes on even further with the increase diagnosis of cancer, Parkinson's, Alzheimer's, depression and infertility. "What an extraordinary achievement for a civilization: to have developed the one diet that reliably makes its people sick!" (Michael Pollen, Food Rules: An Eater's Manual, Penguin Books 2009).

Foods included in the Paleo Free Diet

- Fruit

- Vegetables

- Lean Meat

- Seafood

- Nuts/Seeds

- Healthy Fats (eg. coconut, avocado, nuts and seeds, olive oil, grass fed butter)

Foods NOT included in the Paleo Free Diet

- Dairy

- Grain

- Processed Food

Why not grain?

You may be surprised to see that grains are not included in the Paleo Free Diet. We are accustomed to grains being a part of a balanced diet. However, our bodies are not designed to deal with the nutritional components of grains such as gluten, lectin, and phytates.

Gluten is a protein substance found in wheat, barley and rye. Many people are discovering that their bodies are gluten sensitive and are eliminating gluten from their diet. The most extreme case of gluten sensitivity is Celiac Disease. Individuals with this disease can pick up the minutest trace of gluten and react immediately.

Lectin binds to insulin receptors and can also cause leptin resistance.

Phytates cause minerals to become unavailable during digestion.

Why is dairy a problem?

When purchasing milk, you need to be mindful of the source.

Check out the rest of this book on Amazon

Or go to: http://amzn.to/1jIJUFX

Sugar Detox Guide Beginners

Lose Weight Quickly, Achieve Optimal Health, Feel Energized and Eliminate Sugar Cravings Naturally

Emma Rose

Table of Contents

Introduction   1

The Problem with Too Much Sugar...   5

How do You Know you're Addicted to Sugar?   9

Why? How Do You Get Addicted?   13

How Do Detox Works? Why Detox?   15

How to Start Detox?   19

Some Sugar-Free Recipes   23

Conclusion   37

Preview of Next Book   39

Check Out My Other Books   45

Introduction

I want to thank you and congratulate you for purchasing the book, *"**Sugar Detox Guide for Beginners**: Lose Weight Quickly, Achieve Optimal Health, Feel Energized and Eliminate Sugar Cravings Naturally"*.

This book contains proven steps and strategies on how to detoxify your body and kick Sugar Addiction in the butt within 21 days.

Because of the way food is processed nowadays, most people don't know that almost everything they eat has lots of sugar in it. And with sugar being discovered as the real cause of obesity, heart disease and other illnesses, this is a very bad thing.

Understand Sugar Addiction, its symptoms and the detrimental health effects it has. Know exactly what sugar does to your brain and body. And most importantly, know how exactly you can kick your sugar addiction goodbye!

All my life I've had a sweet tooth. I would even go as far as to say that I had a sugar addiction! Over the last few years my sugar addiction got worse: I had dessert multiple times a day and every day (I guess being a Foods teacher didn't help much). I would joke with people by telling them that I had my servings of vegetables for the day in chocolate...except, I still didn't have the vegetables. It got pretty bad. I knew I hated eating that much dessert but I couldn't stop. I would eat one Ferrero Rochers and then go back for another. As I walked back to the treats, I would pass the mirror and think to myself, "I don't need to have this chocolate. But, ah, what the heck, I don't care." In the end, I'd have about 6

Ferrero Rochers in addition to the other treats I had earlier that day.

Finally, I had to take the huge tray of Ferrero Rochers to school to give to my students on Valentine's Day. There was no way I could eat the other 30 myself. Eating all this sugar caused a huge war within me. I knew that my extreme sugar eating was unhealthy for me but I didn't want to stop. I loved it too much. As a result, I wrestled between the ideal of where I wanted to be and the reality of where I was. I knew I had the discipline to say no to other things, so why couldn't I say no to chocolate?

I eventually came to the point where I was starting to get fed up with not feeling well. I had a lot of chronic pain in my neck and I was constantly tired. I knew that sugar was irritating the problem and causing inflammation in my body. At was starting to reach the breaking point. Ultimately, I chose to go off of sugar for at least three weeks to break the habit I had created for myself. It was seriously a miracle to stay consistent with my goal because I really didn't want to give up my favorite desserts.

I encourage you to make that switch to healthier and happier lifestyle. Cutting out all the processed foods and going back to the basics really does clear up the body and help it function better. I've seen the changes in my own life as hard as it's been to make those changes. You, too, can make the changes necessary and still have your sweets along the way!

Thanks again for purchasing this book, I hope you enjoy it! Please take some time to stop by and LIKE our Facebook page:

https://www.facebook.com/joypublishing

With gratitude,

Emma Rose

Chapter 1

The Problem with Too Much Sugar...

For years, nutritionist have pinned all the caution warning on fats and other additives found in everyone's diets. But the real cause of all the obesity and other complications have been uncovered from the role it plays to weaken your diet and your body.

- *Sugar has no essential nutrients and spells trouble for your teeth.*

  A lot of sugar additives have high levels of calories with literally no essential nutrients, which is why they are called the Empty Calories. When it is said that there are no essential nutrients, it means no proteins, fats, vitamins or minerals, all that is in sugar is just pure energy. If the amount of sugar in your calorie intake goes up to 10 or 20 percent, you'll start having problems in nutrient deficiencies and more.

  Also, being a substance of easily convertible energy, it means that it is not only your body that gets a boost, so does the bad bacteria in your mouth. That could be a major disaster for your teeth. It feeds the bacteria so they multiply faster, harming your mouth (and body) faster.

- *Fructose can overload your liver.*

Sugar is broken down into two simple sugar compounds before it enters the bloodstream. These are fructose and glucose. Glucose can be found in every living cell in all organisms. If you don't consume enough of it from your foods, your body would provide it for you. Now the problematic one is fructose. It is not naturally occurring in your body so you can only get it through your diet. Your body does not really need fructose in order to function properly, but it does taste good.

Fructose is not inherently bad because we do get it from eating fruits, but the only organ that can metabolize it properly is the liver, and it stores the processed fructose as glycogen until your body needs it. Now, if the liver is already full of glycogen, it will transform the rest of the fructose (if you keep on digesting too much) into fat. And this can turn into a fatty-liver problem.

This is usually not a problem who are physically active. Healthy, active people metabolize their fructose faster before it can become a burden to their bodies. This is compared to people who have a sedentary lifestyle who ingest the same high-calorie, high-sugar diet.

- *Sugar can cause insulin resistance that can drive towards diabetes.*

We know that insulin helps the cells focus on burning glucose instead of fat when blood sugar enters these cells. Insulin resistance is caused by the insulin hormone stopping from working properly. Too much glucose in the blood is very toxic and causes the complications of diabetes, like going blind.

When the cells become resistant to insulin, the glucose stacks up in them and contributes to the onset of diseases. These may include obesity, metabolic syndrome, cardiovascular diseases and most commonly, diabetes (type II). Large amounts of sugar consumed have always been associated with insulin resistance.

- *Sugar has fat-promoting effects.*

  Different food types have different effects on the brain and hormones, particularly those that deal with controlling the appetite. Glucose and fructose have opposite effects on the satiation of hunger.

  In a certain medical study, those who drank fructose-sweetened beverages actually become hungrier while those sweetened with glucose got lowered levels of the hunger hormone, Ghrelin. Sugar can provide energy, but it cannot remove hunger, thus this contributes to an increase in calorie intake.

- *Sugar is highly addictive.*

  Sugar causes massive releases of dopamine in the brain. This is like your brain rewarding the body for something it likes. Because of this, people susceptible to addiction become hooked to sugary foods as well as junk foods.

The problem in the saying "Everything in Moderation" is it does not work for people addicted to sugar. The only thing that will help with this true addiction is to completely remove sugars from your diet.

- *It's the sugar and not the fat that raises the cholesterol and contributes to heart disease.*

The world has always blamed saturated fats for heart diseases, which by the way, is the leading cause of death in the world. But, newer studies show that it is not fat but fructose that causes harm to the body's metabolism and thus contribute to diseases. That does not mean that fructose is inherently bad, only that the massive doses of fructose takes a toll on the body over time. After all, fructose is used in just about everything nowadays, especially sweetened beverages and processed food.

It has been proven that stacking up sugar in the blood and cells can raise the small, dense LDL and oxidized LDL triglycerides (also known as very bad stuff!) within mere weeks. And at the same time, the built up fructose also raise blood sugar, insulin levels and abdominal obesity. And this all spell risks for heart diseases.

Chapter 2

How Do You Know You're Addicted to Sugar?

Addiction to sugar is associated to a persistent imbalance in the blood sugar, letting the body show signs and symptoms for the condition. Here are a few observed behavioral and physiological signs that you've become addicted to sugar:

- You have a craving for bread products, sugary beverages, or sweets. This is the most common and easily discernible symptom, so keep watch.

- You have what they call the food coma. It is the feeling of drowsiness and fatigue after a heavy meal. It has always been attributed to eating too much, but now we know that this is the body trying to deal with the sugar influx.

- When you miss a meal, you get a feeling of lightheadedness. Sometimes, you might even feel faint and dizzy, with the accompanying sense of irritation because of bright lights (or even just regular light). If your body gets used to a high energy, high calorie intake every time, missing a meal can make your body go into withdrawal.

- When, after you eat some sweets you get a craving for more. Actually, you feel the craving more once you've eaten the sweets. This is because the fructose in the sugar, by encouraging production of ghrelin, increases the feeling of hunger. This makes for a good appetizer and a bad snack.

- You have become dependent on caffeine to get your body started. You keep looking for coffee and sodas in order to stay awake and keep going.

- You have hard time losing weight; more so than average people. This is not because of your genes and definitely not from being too fat. This is your body being too busy dealing with all that sugar to actually start burning fat.

Usually, these can be alleviated or even completely removed by balancing your blood sugar. Here are the tried and tested methods to do just that:

- Eat more proteins. Protein promotes muscle-building which can help to metabolize your excess fats. For this, you have to ensure that you are digesting them properly. You can check this by monitoring the levels of your stomach acids.

- Eliminate sugar and carbohydrates from your diet. They are good for instant energy but bad for your sugar addiction. Eating regular, healthy meals regularly should be sufficient for your energy needs.

- Eat more good fats, complex carbohydrates, fiber and essential nutrients. A craving for sugar can come from your body not getting enough nutrients. Fiber-rich foods are also great for detoxifying your body not only from the build-up of sugar, but also from fats and other toxins.

- Detoxify your body from sugar!

  It may prove to be a challenge at first, but doing the detox will definitely fix your blood sugar imbalance. And it will set up the stage for an opportunity to fix all other flaws in your diet.

It is reported that sugar addiction is even worse than other kinds of addiction. You might find that it is more difficult to get over, since there is sugar in almost everything you eat and drink, but once you have decided, and you successfully keep at it for these three weeks, you'll see results that you will be proud of.

Chapter 3

Why? How Do You Get Addicted?

It is estimated that sugar is around eight times more addictive than cocaine. Most people would have you think that sugar addiction is just a psychological eating disorder, or that it is just caused by your emotional state. That is not the case. It is a biological addiction, a disorder of the hormones and an error in the chemical balance in your body that causes cravings for sugars and carbohydrates. This will lead to uncontrollable binge eating. There has been a recent study showing that a high-sugar drink has the same addictive effect to the brain as a food-product spiked with cocaine or even morphine.

Most people would not notice that they have a full-blown sugar addiction. This is because they don't know that sugar is in everything that they eat. There was even an event where nutritionists requested food manufacturers to decrease the amount of sugar incorporated into their processed food by 30% to stop an incoming wave of diseases. Nobody reacted to the announcement because the idea was deemed absurd. What? There is sugar in a can of tomato soup? Actually, there is at least four teaspoons of sugar in each serving of that stuff.

When digesting sugar, your brain releases a kind of hormone that gives a wave of good feeling. And at the same time, that feeling activates the addiction center in the brain. Your body, liking the reaction from the stuff, will make you want more and more of it. Since sugar can be found in most food items available, you'll end up overeating, risking ingesting too much of both sugar and carbohydrates than what can be good for your body.

By developing a habit of having a constant high level of sugar in your blood, your body slowly gets used to this diet. Once you miss a meal or when you try to lower your blood sugar, your body then rejects the change. This is what happens when you experience "sugar withdrawal". Many would just use this excuse to eat more sugary sweets. But you have to see that it will only feel horrible at first. Slowly getting your diet back on the right track is worth the trouble.

Chapter 4

How Do Detox Works? Why Detox?

The detoxification works by over-correcting your body's sugar balance. This is done by completely removing sugars from your diet for a period of time to clear out any of the excess sugars before letting you return to your regular (not the sugary-regular, just regular) diet. This process can make you experience some effect that people call "Sugar Withdrawal Syndrome" that may last from a few days to a week. Mostly, it would be better to just muster up all your will power to get over these symptoms, since it will fade as you go along with the detox program. For those experiencing especially serious withdrawal symptoms, physical activity and drinking a lot of water every day will help a lot to ease the conditions. This will also include drinking water when you do feel the huge waves of food/sugar cravings that will attack you through the entire process.

So if the withdrawal can get unpleasant, why detox? Firstly, feeling worse about it actually means you are really getting better and that your body is getting rid of the built up sugar in your blood. Most of all, there are more benefits to sugar detox than just decreasing or removing your excessive craving for sweets. Some of these pluses are:

- You will begin to lose fat faster and easier. You might even find that your body's fat has gone down during the detox.

- You will feel less bloated. It is a feeling attributed to the time during or after a meal. Sugar imbalance also gives the bloated feeling that can persist throughout the day.

- Your tastes will return to normal. That would mean that healthier food will taste better since your sense is not tuned to preferring sweetness anymore. It is like removing your taste buds' bias towards sweet things. You'll be able to enjoy different kinds of food more.

- Your skin will appear clearer. Sugary diets zap out the collagen in your skin, making your complexion look blotchy and pallid. After detox, since you've lessened the sugar and increased water intake, you'll find that your skin has become better-looking than ever.

- You'll have more control over your hunger. After the detox process, you will see that you no longer have random attacks of cravings for sugar, or other food, for that matter.

- You'll have more energy and you'll feel it consistently throughout your day. There will be no more noon times after lunch spent being drowsy.

- You will have a more regular bowel movement. This is seen in detox diets that focus on removing excess sugar and carbs, promoting fiber and other essential nutrients in the process.

- Your attitude might improve, with less depressed moments and a general elevation of mood. Although this mostly comes from the knowledge that you are doing what is good for your body.

- You will definitely lower your body cholesterol; in fact, it would be great to combine this sugar detox program with physical exercise.

- You'll sleep better. A healthy diet usually helps create better sleeping habits.

Other than these physical and behavioral improvements, this sugar detox will also let you have a happier and healthier outlook on life that will help you set up the stage for creating the lifestyle that you have always wanted. Create a goal of making a lifestyle that will let you live longer, healthier, and happier!

Chapter 5

How to Start Detox?

There are basically three things you need to do during the sugar detox period. There are more to it like good exercise and removing other unhealthy diets as well. But for now these are the things you have to focus on:

1. You have to avoid eating or drinking all sugar and simple carbohydrates from your diet for 21 days, uninterrupted. There is a very long list of things you cannot eat compared to the much shorter one of recommended food. You must follow these at all times.

2. You have to watch what you eat for those three weeks. It would be recommended to keep a food journal for this task. Doing so will make it easier for you to watch out what you eat and you'll find it easier to control eating impulses. It can even encourage you to continue the food journal even after the detox period. You might also want to include a computation of your total calorie intake for each entry.

3. If you missed a day of detoxification or if you slip up and eat something you're not supposed to even just once (eating or drinking something with sugar or simple carbs), you'll have to start from zero. This will motivate you to try hurdling through the 21 days without returning to day one.

Before you do start the sugar detox process, you have to consider some of these things in your mind. But, just a warning:

you have to hold steadfast. Remember what they say about beauty and health, "no pain, no gain". Not that you'll be in pain, for the most part. Here are some of the things you need to think about:

- *21 Days can feel like an eternity.*

  You may have chosen this detox plan on a whim. Maybe you just saw it in a forum or you heard someone who did well with it. Well, you'll see 21 days solidly spent on this detox is no walk in the park. It's going to be like crawling through briars in the middle of a thunderstorm. You have to keep your determination steadfast and just don't be discouraged because it will definitely prove to be a challenge. The rewards will all be worth it in the end, that's for sure.

- *You'll have to stick to it honestly.*

  Finishing your 21-day sugar detox within less than 21 days will be the easiest way to relapse into our sugar addiction. Cutting your diet plan this way will ensure the return of your problematic habit, probably more strongly than before. It is a carefully-made program that will ensure ridding both your body and your mind of the uncontrollable craving for sugar. So, just because you feel a little better after a week or two, you cannot just cut the detox process that short. It is set at 21 days for a reason.

  Absolutely don't cheat, shortcut or mess it up. If you did, even by the tiniest little bit, restart and do it properly for three weeks.

- *A one-time 3-week detox may not be enough.*

  If you think a single three-week detox will work for you, don't be too sure. A lifetime worth of sugar addiction can take quite a few passes of this detox process to completely clear out. Advice: keep at it until you've been completely "cured" of the built up sugar over all those years. But do remember to take a break. Say after three weeks of uninterrupted detox, return to a normal (albeit a healthier) diet and then restart after some time following through the three weeks again.

- *It is not a lifestyle changing plan.*

  It is just the tip of the ice berg, so to say. You have to decide what lifestyle you would be following after your detox. That is because you will definitely have to leave the high-carb, high-sugar lifestyle you've had before, so take a note of this. You can even use this opportunity to fix more than just your diet in your lifestyle. After all, it will be easier for you to change some of your unhealthy habits when you don't have those persistent cravings anymore. But note that this will just be a start if you want a complete lifestyle change.

- *It is adjustable to fit different individuals.*

  Definitely better than most of the unchangeable diet programs, sugar detox can take form on different levels or intensity to suit your sugar use. There are some designed for those who have flat-out sugar addiction. While there is also some plans that is preferred by the ones who don't consume that much sugar, there are those that are made for slow-starters. Either that or it is because they feel that the higher level detox programs are too much. Being a bit uncomfortable with the designed plan is normal; you are trying to change your habits after all. But you should know that too much discomfort is detrimental to your progress. So, choose a detox plan that will suit your requirements.

- *The detox process pushes all the bad things out. It will let you feel in full what all that sugar was doing to your body.*

You will definitely feel the effects of withdrawal. The worst of the effects of that built up sugar in your body will certainly show themselves during the process. Remember to keep your determination to help you overcome these things and the experiences that will obstruct the path of your detoxification in the first few days.

Your nutritionist or physician can suggest further additions to this diet as well as other things you can do to make it more effective. They can give helpful advice such as the kind of physical activity you can maintain during the detox period. If you didn't want to consult with a doctor, you can find many references on the subject. There are many discussions about tried and tested diet plans in books, articles and blogs online.

Chapter 6

Some Sugar-free Recipes

Here are some of the food products you would want to have in your diet during the sugar detox program:

- Herbs

- Vegetables (except potatoes)

- Beans

- Avocado

- Carrots

- Coconut Oil

- Eggs

- Fish

- Meat

- Nuts

- Olive Oil

- Seed-foods

- Tomatoes

- Citrus Fruits (not the sweet citrus ones though)

- Unsweetened chocolate (Dark and black chocolates are actually good for you. Even if they're quite bitter, they can substitute desserts. It is an acquired taste after all so they might take a little getting used to.)

And the stuff you need to avoid:

- Alcohol

- Flour and flour-based products

- Fried food

- Fruit juices

- Artificial sweeteners (they're worse than sugar, promise!)

- fruits

- Bread products

- Corn syrup (start checking labels, this stuff is in many things)

- Candy

- honey

- Cereal

- Maple syrup

- Cheese

- Potatoes (yes, even fries)

- Dairy products

- oatmeal

- Cream sauces

- Sugar

- Soy

- Tortillas and other corn-based crackers

- White rice

- Trans-fat (these should be in the label, look them up)

- Yogurt (even the non-fat, unsweetened ones!)

- Pasta (all of them)

- Pizza

Meatballs in Tomato Sauce

Ingredients:

- ¼ cup Parmesan cheese
- 2 lightly beaten eggs
- 1/3 cup whole wheat bread crumbs
- 12 oz. or 3 pieces sausages removed from casings
- 1 lb. ground beef (choose one with less fat)
- 1 tsp. minced garlic
- Salt
- Pepper
- Parmesan cheese for garnish

Sauce:
- 1 tbsp. minced garlic
- 2 cans tomatoes, diced and pureed
- 1 tsp. dried oregano
- 2 tsp. dried basil
- salt

Procedure:

1. Preheat the oven to 425° F. Remove the sausages and ground beef from the cold. Squeeze the sausage meat from their casings and bring both meats to room temperature.

2. Put the bread crumbs in a bowl and add 1/3 cup of hot water. Let the crumbs absorb the water before adding the garlic, salt, pepper, grated Parmesan cheese and the eggs. After mixing them well, add the meats and use your hands to combine them.

3. Prepare the pan or dish with oil or nonstick spray. Round up meatballs with your hands, using a spoon to measure out the meat. Arrange them so they'll have space between each meatball.

4. Puree the tomatoes. After putting it in a bowl, add in the salt, herbs and garlic. Pour this sauce over the meatballs. Sprinkle the remaining cheese over them. Bake them until the sauce and the cheese is bubbling. That would take just over half an hour.

Serve it hot with more Parmesan sprinkled on the meatballs.

This recipe makes about 6 servings.

Chicken Nuggets with Almonds

Ingredients:

- 2 tbsp. olive oil
- 1 tsp. paprika
- ½ cup almond flour or almond meal
- ½ tsp. chicken seasoning
- 2 skinless chicken breasts, boneless

Procedure:

1. Preheat oven to 400° F. Prepare the pan and baking sheet with the olive oil.

2. Remove all tendons and visible fat from the chicken then cut it into nuggets (each breast piece should make about 5 pieces). Make sure they are all of the same thickness, using a kitchen mallet to even out differences.

3. Combine the rest of the ingredients in a bowl and mix well. Dip each nugget into this mixture, making sure it coats the chicken evenly. Line them up into the pan with the baking sheet.

4. Cook for around 10 minutes, until the side touching the pan is slightly browned. The nuggets become too hard and chewy when overcooked so don't overdo it. Once one side is cooked, turn the nuggets and then cook for another 10 minutes.

5. Serve hot with your favorite chicken nugget dip.

This recipe makes about 2 servings.

Muffin Pan Meal

Ingredients:

- 6 eggs
- 8 ½ oz. muffin mix (or corn bread)
- Salt
- Pepper
- 15 oz. corned beef

Procedure:

1. Grease the 12-cup muffin pan. Divide the corned beef into six of these cups. Press them down, so that it sticks to the bottom and comes up at the sides to form shells.

2. Break an egg into each shell and season with some salt and pepper.

3. Prepare muffin mix according to the instructions on the packaging. Spoon the muffin batter into the remaining 6 cups.

4. Bake at 400° F for up to 20 minutes or just when the muffins are golden brown.

5. Put the cooked egg and shell onto the muffins as toppings. Serve immediately. They could also be reheated by putting them through the microwave for a few seconds on mid-level heat.

This recipe makes 4 - 6 servings.

Chicken Skillet

Ingredients:

- 3 tbsp. olive oil
- ½ chopped green pepper
- 1 chopped onion
- 4 crushed garlic cloves
- 1 ½ lbs. boneless chicken
- Salt
- Pepper

Procedure:

1. Slice the chicken to your desired serving pieces.

2. Heat the oil in the skillet and cook the chicken until they are nearly done.

3. Add the garlic, onion and the green pepper, sauté them with the chicken.

4. You know you are finished cooking when the chicken is slightly browned and the onion has become soft.

5. After that, you can add some choice vegetables and sauté until cooked to your liking.

6. Season with salt and pepper.

Beef Barbecue Sandwiches and Burritos

Ingredients:

- Hamburger buns
- 1 packet taco seasoning
- Flour tortillas with your favorite toppings
- 1 bottle of barbecue sauce
- 5 lbs. roast beef

Procedure:

1. Shred well-cooked roast meat with a fork. Reserve half of the meat for the sandwiches. Drain any liquid left in the pot with the meat. Put the taco seasoning and stir in two cups of water with the remaining half of the meat. Cook until heated through.

2. Serve on tortillas.

3. Take the other half and stir in the barbecue sauce. Heat mixture in the microwave (or on a stove top).

4. Serve on buns.

This recipe makes about 4 servings.

Onion Rings

Ingredients:

- 2 onions, choose the white ones
- ½ red pepper powder or chili powder
- 1 tsp. ground black pepper
- Salt
- 250 ml beer
- 1 ¾ cup flour
- ¼ cup corn meal

Procedure:

1. Mix the flour and corn meal, stirring in the red and black pepper, salt and beer. Make sure all the ingredients are mixed evenly. Afterwards, cover it and let it sit for an hour.

2. In a pan, heat about 5 cm-high peanut or olive oil until it is around 370° F.

3. On a plate filled with a mound of flour, toss 5 or 6 pieces of onion rings, and then dip it in your prepared batter. Drop them one at a time into the oil.

4. Cook the rings for a few minutes until they are sufficiently browned on both sides. Drain off all oil with paper towels or by putting them on a wire rack. Salt the rings and serve hot.

This recipe makes 4-6 servings.

Eggplant Sticks

Ingredients:

- ½ cup beaten eggs
- ¾ tsp. garlic and salt powder
- 1 cup spaghetti sauce or tomato sauce of your choice
- 1 eggplant (1 ¼ lbs.)
- Seasoning of your choice

Procedure:

1. Cut eggplant into snack-sized sticks.

2. In a long bowl or on a dish, combine the garlic and salt powder, with your choice seasoning. Dip each eggplant stick into the beaten eggs then coat it in the powder mixture. Arrange them on a baking sheet.

3. Spray the laid out sticks with cooking spray. Broil the sticks for 3 minutes. Remove the baking sheet from the oven afterwards.

4. Turn the sticks and spritz them again with the cooking spray. Cook for another 2 minutes or when they are browned to your liking.

5. Serve hot. Prepare the tomato sauce as your dip.

This recipe makes about 8 servings.

Sausage Snacks

Ingredients:

- 12 oz. spicy pork sausages, ground
- 12 oz. pork sausages, ground
- Ham slices
- Scrambled eggs, fried
- mayonnaise

Procedure:

1. Preheat your broiler.

2. Mix and cook the ground pork sausage and the spicy ground pork sausage in a well-oiled skillet. Brown the ground pork over medium high heat. Drain the sausage of any liquid.

3. Process the ground pork with the mayonnaise until they are incorporated well.

4. On each ham slice, place some of the ground pork mixture and some scrambled eggs. Roll them up and secure with a toothpick.

5. Broil the rolls for 3 to 5 minutes. Check it frequently, and finishing when they are sufficiently toasted.

This recipe makes about 5-6 servings.

Roasted Chickpeas

Ingredients:

- Olive oil or cooking spray
- Salt
- 1 tsp. chili powder
- 1 tsp. paprika
- 1 tsp. coriander
- 1 tsp. cumin
- 1 tsp. garlic powder
- 1 tsp. curry powder

Procedure:

1. Preheat oven to 375° F. Drain chickpeas and let them completely dry. If you need to, you can pat dry them with a paper towel.

2. Arrange them on a baking sheet, laying them on a single layer. Roast for around half an hour, shaking the pan every ten minutes. Just make sure they don't burn. You'll know they are done when they have turned golden brown with crunchy insides instead of moist.

3. Combine all the spices in a bowl, mixing them well. Remove the chickpeas from the oven when they are done and spray them with olive oil.

4. Toss the chickpeas with the spices while they're still hot.

5. They are preferably served hot. But you can also let them cool in room temperature and then place them in airtight Ziploc bags afterwards.

This recipe makes about 3 servings.

Conclusion

Thank you again for purchasing *"**Sugar Detox Guide for Beginners**: Lose Weight Quickly, Achieve Optimal Health, Feel Energized and Eliminate Sugar Cravings Naturally"*!

I hope this book was able to help you to have a less-sugary diet and have a more positive outlook to set you up for a good and healthy lifestyle.

The next step is to create a new lifestyle that will let you live healthier and happier.

Finally, if you enjoyed this book, please take the time to share your thoughts and post a review on Amazon. It'd be greatly appreciated!

I would love for you to share your experiences, stories and encouragements with me. My email address is emmarosekindle@gmail.com

In addition, please remember to check out our Facebook page in order to find other resources and upcoming promotions:

https://www.facebook.com/joypublishing

With sincere thanks,

Emma Rose

Emma Rose

Preview of "Clean Eating Guide: Lose Weight Quickly, Achieve Optimal Health and Feel Energized with Clean Eating for Busy Families and Clean Eating Recipes

Introduction

I want to thank you and congratulate you for purchasing the book, *"Clean Eating Guide: Lose Weight Quickly, Achieve Optimal Health and Feel Energized with Clean Eating For Busy Families and Clean Eating Recipes"*.

This book contains proven steps and strategies on how to lose weight, have more energy, and stay healthy using the principles of clean eating.

There are so many different kinds of diet programs and products available in the market today and all you need to do is choose the one that you think will work best for you. If you do not want to try new products that helps you lose weight and boosts your energy, you should stick to something more basic and natural such as clean eating.

In this book, you will learn everything you need to know about clean eating. It is important to find out everything you can about this type of diet before you incorporate it in your lifestyle. You will learn about the benefits and principles of clean eating and some useful tips that can help you along the way. This book also includes some easy recipes that promote clean eating.

Thanks again for purchasing this book, I hope you enjoy it! Please take some time to stop by and LIKE our Facebook page:

https://www.facebook.com/joypublishing

With gratitude,

Emma Rose

Chapter 1

What Is Clean Eating?

You have probably come across the term 'clean eating' but you are still not familiar about its exact meaning. This is being used by people who work in the health and fitness industry such as personal trainers ad dietitians. People who are health conscious and workout fanatic also often use this word. Does it have something to do with cleaning the food before eating or cooking? Or maybe it has something to do with the kind of food that you eat.

The loose definition of clean eating is eating food in its most natural state. These days, people are starting to pay more attention to the kinds of food that they eat and how these foods are made. They take note of the food's ingredients and make sure that the food product only contains all natural ingredients.

The term clean eating first came out in the 1990s. Today, it is still being used by health conscious individuals from different backgrounds and culture to refer to the kind of all natural diet that they have. The definition of clean eating can vary from person to person. Some define clean eating as eating mostly fruits and vegetables while others define it as not eating anything artificial. You will find out more about these things as you read this book.

What Clean Eating is not?

If you think clean eating is another diet program, like the South Beach diet or Paleo diet, you are wrong because clean eating is a way of life. It also does not follow any strict rules about what food group to eat and not to eat, how many calories you should consume in a meal, and so on. This is the most basic way of healthy eating that promotes weight loss and boost energy. Everybody can do this, even those who are not trying to lose weight.

Clean eating will not make you feel deprived or frustrated because it is so easy to follow. You do not even need to have a really strong determination because it is all a matter of choosing natural over artificial.

Is there such a thing as 'dirty' eating?

You are probably wondering if there is such a thing as 'dirty' eating or the opposite of clean eating. Clean eating does not literally mean eating foods that have less dirt. It means that you are choosing the best and healthiest food choices from different food groups in their most natural state. 'Dirty' eating is not the opposite of clean eating because there is no such thing as eating dirty. The opposite of clean eating is choosing the wrong food to eat and eating junk foods and processed foods that leave toxins in your body.

Clean eating also looks at the source of food. It should not come from large commercial manufacturers that use machines to process food. The foods that clean eaters usually use come from small farms that do not use chemicals and undergo processes. This is why clean eating is often associated with organic eating.

Check out the rest of "Clean Eating Guide: Lose Weight Quickly, Achieve Optimal Health and Feel Energized with Clean Eating for Busy Families and Clean Eating Recipes" on Amazon

Or go to: http://amzn.to/UVzNER

Check Out My Other Books

Below you'll find some of my other books also available on Amazon and Kindle. Search for these titles on the Amazon website to find them.

Paleo Free Diet Guide for Beginners: Over 50 Paleo Free Recipes for Optimal Health & Fast Weight Loss

Paleo Desserts: Satisfy Your Sweet Tooth With Over 100 Quick & Easy Paleo Dessert Recipes & Paleo Baking Recipes

Raw Food Diet Guide: Lose Weight Quickly, Achieve Optimal Health & Feel Energized with the Raw Food Diet & Raw Food Recipes

Clean Eating Guide: Lose Weight Quickly, Achieve Optimal Health & Feel Energized with Clean Eating For Busy Families & Clean Eating Recipes

Alkaline Diet Guide: Lose Weight Quickly, Achieve Optimal Health & Feel Energized with the Alkaline Diet & Alkaline Recipes

Coconut Flour Recipes for Optimal Health & Quick Weight Loss: Gluten Free Recipes for Celiac Disease, Gluten Sensitivities & Paleo Free Diets

Almond Flour Recipes for Optimal Health & Quick Weight Loss: Gluten Free Recipes for Celiac Disease, Gluten Sensitivities & Paleo Free Diets

Wheat Free Diet for Beginners: Lose Weight Quickly, Achieve Optimal Health & Feel Energized with Gluten Free Recipes for Celiac Disease, Gluten Sensitivities & Paleo Free Diets

Detox Diet Guide: Lose Weight Quickly, Achieve Optimal Health & Feel Energized Through the 10 Day Detox

Sugar Detox Guide for Beginners: Lose Weight Quickly, Achieve Optimal Health, Feel Energized & Eliminate Sugar Cravings Naturally

Ketogenic Diet Guide for Beginners: How to Achieve Rapid Weight Loss, Optimal Health & Unstoppable Energy with Ketogenic Diet Recipes

Anti Inflammatory Diet for Beginners: Lose Weight Fast, Optimize Health, Slow Aging, Fight Inflammation, Conquer Pain & Increase Energy with the Anti Inflammation Diet Recipes

www.ingramcontent.com/pod-product-compliance
Lightning Source LLC
Chambersburg PA
CBHW060512290526
45791CB00001B/364